THE FACILITATOR GUIDE FOR

Core Competencies of Civility
in nursing & healthcare

Cynthia Clark, PhD, RN, ANEF, FAAN
Jessica G. Smith, PhD, RN

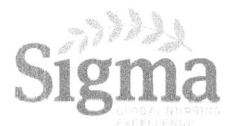

Copyright © 2023 by Sigma Theta Tau International Honor Society of Nursing

All rights reserved. This book is protected by copyright. No part of it may be reproduced, stored in a retrieval system, or transmitted in any form or by any means, electronic, mechanical, photocopying, recording, or otherwise, without written permission from the publisher. Any trademarks, service marks, design rights, or similar rights that are mentioned, used, or cited in this book are the property of their respective owners. Their use here does not imply that you may use them for a similar or any other purpose.

This book is not intended to be a substitute for the medical advice of a licensed medical professional. The author and publisher have made every effort to ensure the accuracy of the information contained within at the time of its publication and shall have no liability or responsibility to any person or entity regarding any loss or damage incurred, or alleged to have incurred, directly or indirectly, by the information contained in this book. The author and publisher make no warranties, express or implied, with respect to its content, and no warranties may be created or extended by sales representatives or written sales materials. The author and publisher have no responsibility for the consistency or accuracy of URLs and content of third-party websites referenced in this book.

Sigma Theta Tau International Honor Society of Nursing (Sigma) is a nonprofit organization whose mission is developing nurse leaders anywhere to improve healthcare everywhere. Founded in 1922, Sigma has more than 135,000 active members in over 100 countries and territories. Members include practicing nurses, instructors, researchers, policymakers, entrepreneurs, and others. Sigma's more than 540 chapters are located at more than 700 institutions of higher education throughout Armenia, Australia, Botswana, Brazil, Canada, Colombia, Croatia, England, Eswatini, Ghana, Hong Kong, Ireland, Israel, Italy, Jamaica, Japan, Jordan, Kenya, Lebanon, Malawi, Mexico, the Netherlands, Nigeria, Pakistan, Philippines, Portugal, Puerto Rico, Scotland, Singapore, South Africa, South Korea, Sweden, Taiwan, Tanzania, Thailand, the United States, and Wales. Learn more at www.sigmanursing.org.

Sigma Theta Tau International
550 West North Street
Indianapolis, IN, USA 46202

To request a review copy for course adoption, order additional books, buy in bulk, or purchase for corporate use, contact Sigma Marketplace at 888.654.4968 (US/Canada toll-free), +1.317.687.2256 (International), or solutions@sigmamarketplace.org.

To request author information, or for speaker or other media requests, contact Sigma Marketing at 888.634.7575 (US/Canada toll-free) or +1.317.634.8171 (International).

ISBN: 9781646480708
PDF ISBN: 9781646480715

First Printing, 2022

Publisher: Dustin Sullivan
Acquisitions Editor: Emily Hatch
Development Editor: Jill Stanley
Cover Designer: Rebecca Batchelor
Interior Design/Page Layout: Rebecca Batchelor
Managing Editor: Carla Hall
Publications Specialist: Todd Lothery
Project Editor: Alexandra Andrzejewski
Copy Editor: Todd Lothery
Proofreader: Todd Lothery

About the Authors

Cynthia Clark, PhD, RN, ANEF, FAAN, is founder of Civility Matters and Professor Emeritus at Boise State University. As a clinician, she specialized in adolescent mental health, substance abuse intervention and recovery, and suicide and violence prevention. She is a leading expert in fostering civility and healthy work environments around the globe. Her groundbreaking work on fostering civility has brought national and international attention to the controversial issues of incivility in academic and work environments. Her theory-driven interventions, empirical measurements, theoretical models, and reflective assessments provide best practices to prevent, measure, and address uncivil behavior and to create healthy workplaces.

Jessica G. Smith, PhD, RN, is an Assistant Professor at the University of Texas at Arlington College of Nursing and Health Innovation. She received her PhD in nursing from the University of Wisconsin-Milwaukee in 2016. She completed a two-year postdoctoral fellowship (2016–2018) at the Center for Health Outcomes and Policy Research at the University of Pennsylvania. Her areas of interest include understanding the needs of the acute rural nurse workforce to deliver safer patient care and how work environments and processes influence nurse well-being.

Table of Contents

1 What Is Civility, and Why Does It Matter? 1
    Before You Begin 2
    Key Concepts 3
    Rationale for Implementation 4
    Application of the Concepts 5
    Reflection 5
    References 6

2 The Detrimental Impact of Workplace Aggression 7
    Before You Begin 8
    Key Concepts 9
    Rationale for Implementation 11
    Application of the Concepts 11
    Reflection 12
    References 13

3 The Power and Imperative of Self-Awareness 15
    Before You Begin 16
    Key Concepts 17
    Rationale for Implementation 18
    Application of the Concepts 19
    Reflection 20
    References 21

4 Practicing the Fundamentals of Civility 23
    Before You Begin 24
    Key Concepts 25
    Rationale for Implementation 26
    Application of the Concepts 26
    Reflection 27
    References 29

5 Honing Communication Skills and Conflict Competence 31
Before You Begin 32
Key Concepts 33
Rationale for Implementation 35
Application of the Concepts 35
Reflection 42
References 42

6 The Power of Leadership, Visioning, and Finding Our WHY ... 45
Before You Begin 46
Key Concepts 47
Rationale for Implementation 48
Application of the Concepts 49
Reflection 50
References 51

7 Optimizing Self-Care and Professional Well-Being 53
Before You Begin 54
Key Concepts 55
Rationale for Implementation 57
Application of the Concepts 58
Reflection 59
References 59

8 Leadership Support and Raising Awareness for Organizational Change 61
Before You Begin 62
Key Concepts 63
Rationale for Implementation 65
Application of the Concepts 65
Reflection 67
References 67

9 Galvanizing a High-Performing Civility Team 69
Before You Begin 70
Key Concepts 72
Rationale for Implementation 74

	Application of the Concepts..................................75
	Reflection 76
	References..77
10	**Develop, Implement, and Evaluate a Data-Driven Action Plan**.....................................**79**
	Before You Begin.....................................80
	Key Concepts..82
	Rationale for Implementation 83
	Application of the Concepts..............................84
	Reflection 85
	References..85
11	**Securing Civility Into the Organizational Culture Through Policy Development** **87**
	Before You Begin.....................................88
	Key Concepts..89
	Rationale for Implementation 92
	Application of the Concepts..............................92
	Reflection 94
	References..94
12	**Celebrating Civility: A Powerful Engine to Uplift and Transform the Profession** **95**
	Before You Begin.....................................96
	Key Concepts..97
	Rationale for Implementation 98
	Application of the Concepts..............................99
	Reflection 100
	References...101

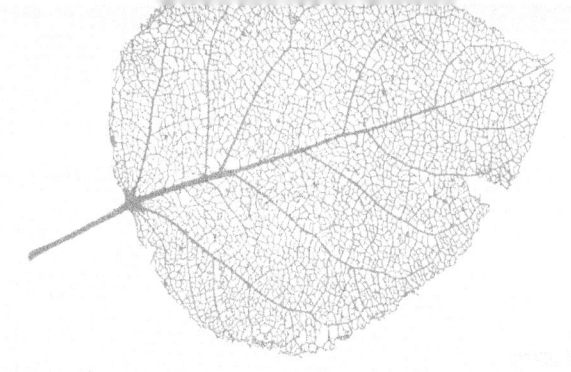

1

What Is Civility, and Why Does It Matter?

LEARNING OUTCOMES

- Define the concept of civility.
- Explain the importance of authentic civility and ethical behavior in nursing and healthcare.
- Illustrate how being civil is a choice.
- Describe concepts of the Conceptual Model for Achieving a Culture of Belonging.
- Understand how diversity, equity, inclusion, and civility relate in nursing and healthcare.
- Identify how life events and experiences impact one's worldview.

Before You Begin

When facilitating discussion on sensitive topics such as civility, incivility, diversity, equity, and inclusion, facilitators must keep an open mind, avoid imposing their personal values and opinions on others, and be comfortable with varying perspectives—especially from learners who may challenge the veracity of the material, express controversial or opposing points of views, or, in some cases, offer hotly contested opinions or protests. Because viewpoints are often based on historical and personal experiences, comments may stem from deeply held beliefs and be accompanied by a range of emotions. Thus, group discussions have the potential to become intense and challenging to facilitate.

To set the stage for productive and meaningful group discussions, facilitators need to clearly identify the purpose of the discussion, remind learners about the importance of respectful communication, review the principles of sound group dynamics, and define expected norms or rules of engagement. Doing so lessens the risk of the learners' experiences and viewpoints being misconstrued, diminished, or devalued. The overall goal is to foster engagement, reflective thinking, and productive discourse so that learners feel safe to express their thoughts and ideas, and, in turn, class members gain greater awareness and a deeper understanding of the topic dimensions.

In this chapter, concepts of civility, diversity, equity, inclusion, and belonging are introduced and discussed. Learner activities include identifying how personal life events and experiences have shaped their worldview and impacted self and others. Exploring this personal inner landscape requires experienced and skilled facilitators to foster a learning environment where everyone feels welcomed, valued, and productive.

When facilitating discussion on these important topics, bear in mind that perceptions of the same concept can vary widely. For example, one might agree that "civility lies in the eye of the beholder." In other words, a behavior perceived to be uncivil by one individual may be perceived as civil by another. Perceptions are shaped by assumed intent, the context in which the behavior occurs, and attitudes and beliefs held by the recipient of the behavior. Because perceptions vary, the intent and interpretation of behaviors need to be consistently examined and questioned.

Let's consider the concept of civility as one example. The true essence of civility—and how civility is portrayed in *Core Competencies of Civility in Nursing & Healthcare*—refers to co-creating a respectful, psychologically safe, and inclusive environment that brings people together. It means fostering an authentic milieu of belonging that rejects civility as a way of silencing voices of disagreement, squelching dissent, or allowing disparities to persist. To illustrate this point, consider the words of Karen Grigsby Bates (2019, para. 3): "For many people of color in the United States, civility isn't so much social lubricant as it is a vehicle for containing them, preventing social mobility, and preserving the status quo." Thus, civility must not become a weapon to maintain the status quo or silence differing points of view.

Clearly, definitions of civility vary. While the pursuit of civility may be a worthy goal, as Zurn (2013) eloquently observed, political civility is a tension-filled ideal that may be misused for nefarious ends such as unjustifiable marginalization and exclusion. Thus, being intentional to include perspectives that are not the voices of the dominant culture models diversity of thought, moves learners from the margins to the center, and demonstrates an openness to multiple points of view (Gannon, 2020).

Key Concepts

After reading the chapter, ask the learners to test their understanding of the concepts with short answers.

1. What is civility?

    Answer: Choosing to engage in a welcoming, respectful, inclusive manner to foster a culture of equity and belonging—to create community and meaningful connections—including during times when we disagree or when opposing views are expressed.

2. Describe the difference between being "merely" civil and "authentically" civil. Then, explain the outcomes of authentic civility.

    Answer: Mere or nominal civility is defined as minimal conformity to norms of respectful behavior, while true or authentic civility means being willing to engage in respectful communication, meaningful social discourse, and constructive conflict. Outcomes of authentic civility include establishment of a civil society, supportive learning environments, positive work environments, optimal patient outcomes, improved relationships, and productive social discourse.

3. Discuss how interacting with civility is a choice.

    Answer: Being civil is a decision we make every day with each encounter and interaction. Civility is being intentional about showing respect for the dignity, perspectives, and well-being of self and others. Civility helps create work and learning environments where all members feel valued and have a sense of belonging, and it helps foster a milieu where inclusion, diversity, and equity thrive.

4. Describe the ethical imperative for civility.

    Answer: The American Nurses Association's (ANA) Code of Ethics for Nurses (2015) states that all nurses have a moral obligation to "create an ethical environment and culture of civility and kindness, treating colleagues, coworkers, employees, students, and others with dignity and respect" (p. 4). The ANA Code of Ethics for Nurses is consistent with the International Council of Nurses' Code of Ethics (2012), emphasizing the nurse's obligation to respect human rights, treat people with dignity and respect, and provide respectful and unrestricted care.

5. What are the concepts of the Conceptual Model for Achieving a Culture of Belonging?

   Answer: Self and other awareness, civility and respect for diversity and human dignity, psychological safety, courageous conversation, authentic connection, community building, diversity, equity, inclusion, and belonging.

6. How do the concepts of the Conceptual Model for Achieving a Culture of Belonging interrelate?

   Answer: Self and other awareness, civility and respect for diversity and human dignity, psychological safety, and courageous conversations form the foundation for an organization whereby diversity, equity, and inclusion thrive and help build and sustain a culture of belonging.

7. What are the definitions of diversity, equity, and inclusion?

   Answer: *Diversity* refers to an organization's mix of people and recognizes the value of every person and every group. Issues of diversity can include race, ethnicity, gender identity, age, national origin, religion, ability, sexual orientation, socioeconomic status, education, marital status, language, physical appearance, and more. *Equity* refers to fair, unbiased treatment, access, and opportunity for all people. Equity includes identifying and removing barriers and obstacles that prevent or impede individuals from fully participating in the organization. *Inclusion* occurs when traditionally excluded individuals or groups are welcomed into processes, activities, and decision-making in a way that shares power.

Rationale for Implementation

After reading the chapter, ask the learners to test their understanding of the concepts with short answers.

1. Why does civility matter in work and learning environments?

   Answer: Civility helps to create work and learning environments where all members feel valued and have a sense of belonging.

2. Why is it important for an organization to foster a culture of belonging?

   Answer: When people have a true sense of belonging, they are more confident in their abilities to authentically represent themselves, express ideas, and share experiences because they know their input is valued.

Application of the Concepts

Working in small groups, instruct learners to complete the following exercise.

1. Group Activity: Understanding the Conceptual Model for Achieving a Culture of Belonging

Imagine that you are a member of a team of nurses or a nursing faculty group charged with improving the culture of your work or learning environment. Working in teams of five to six members, describe your basic understanding of how the Conceptual Model for Achieving a Culture of Belonging might be used to frame the process.

Example answer: First, it is important to self-reflect on your own behaviors, interactions, perspectives, ideas, biases, etc., as well as lead a discussion for other members of the team to self-reflect. Engaging the team in making a genuine commitment to civility and respect for diversity and human dignity helps set the stage for creating psychological safety and providing a safe space for courageous conversation and constructive conflict negotiation. These measures are foundational to building community and authentic connections where diversity, equity, and inclusion thrive, leading to a culture of belonging.

Reflection

Reflection is an integral aspect of learning, involving inquiry, discussion, and problem-solving. In this section, learners are asked to reflect on what they have learned from Chapter 1 by sharing ideas, takeaways, application of information, and thoughtful feedback. Working in small groups, teams, or learning circles is a learner-centered approach designed to inspire collaboration and build synergy by problem-solving together.

1. Think about what civility meant to you before you read this chapter compared to after. Was there anything you learned about civility that you did not consider before? Why or why not? Going forward, how do you see yourself as a member of the healthcare professions fostering a culture of belonging?

2. Using the Civility Reflection provided in Chapter 1, describe how your life events and experiences have impacted your worldview, life, and the lives of others.

    Take a moment to sit in silence and reflect. If you wish, record your thoughts in a journal. Think deeply and introspectively about your childhood and adolescence. Where and when does your story begin? Where did you grow up and go to school? Did you travel to far-off places or stay mainly in your backyard? How have your life events and experiences shaped the person you have become and continue to become? How have these events and experiences impacted your life and the lives of others around you? Who were the most influential people of your childhood? What lessons did you learn? How are the lessons still affecting your life today? If you are inclined, share your story with a trusted friend, family member, or colleague.

Objective: Open personal reflection of the learner's experiences and understanding of civility and how their life experiences have impacted their life, worldview, and the lives of others. These can be evaluated as short reflective essays or used as discussion starters.

References

American Nurses Association. (2015). *The code of ethics for nurses with interpretive statements*. Author.

Gannon, K. M. (2020). *Radical hope: A teaching manifesto*. West Virginia University Press.

Grigsby Bates, K. (March 14, 2019). *When civility is used as a cudgel against people of color*. All Things Considered, National Public Radio. https://www.npr.org/sections/codeswitch/2019/03/14/700897826/when-civility-is-used-as-a-cudgel-against-people-of-color

International Council of Nurses. (2012). *The ICN code of ethics for nurses*. https://www.icn.ch/sites/default/files/inline-files/2012_ICN_Codeofethicsfornurses_%20eng.pdf

Zurn, C. F. (2013). Political civility: Another illusionistic ideal. *Public Affairs Quarterly, 27*(4), 341–368. http://www.jstor.org/stable/43575586

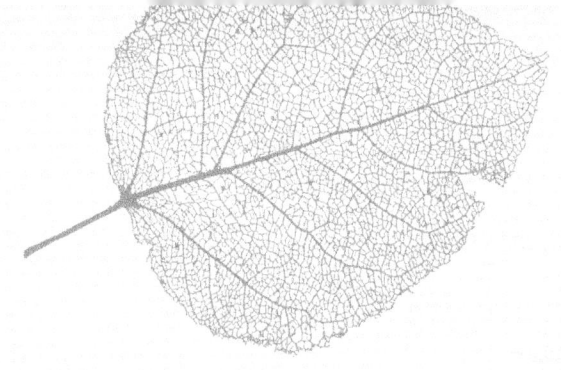

2

The Detrimental Impact of Workplace Aggression

> ### LEARNING OUTCOMES
>
> - Describe the impact of workplace aggression in healthcare for patients, healthcare workers, nursing educators, nursing students, and new nurses.
>
> - Using the Continuum of Workplace Aggression, describe the impact of unaddressed lower-level forms of aggression that can occur in the workplace.
>
> - Define the different forms of workplace violence according to the National Institute for Occupational Safety & Health.
>
> - Identify barriers to addressing workplace aggression.

Before You Begin

Chapter 2 provides a deepened and empirical understanding of the myriad forms of incivility and workplace aggression. The detrimental impact of these aggressions is well documented, and much has been written about their negative effects on individuals, teams, organizations, and patient care. Before you begin facilitating the content contained in Chapter 2, consider doing some additional background reading. For example, if you are unfamiliar with various behaviors depicted on the Continuum of Workplace Aggression, avail yourself of some of the readings provided in the reference list for Chapter 2. You might also consider cofacilitating this content with another colleague experienced with teaching content illustrated on the continuum and described in the chapter. Be aware of your own feelings regarding the various types of aggressions discussed in Chapter 2, especially if they bring up painful memories. Sharing and debriefing your experiences with a trusted colleague before facilitating class can be a helpful exercise.

This chapter contains graphic descriptions of workplace aggression, and facilitators are wise to anticipate a range of feelings and responses from learners. It is important to create a safe learning environment where learners are encouraged to describe workplace aggressions they have either experienced or witnessed and to provide them with opportunities to express their feelings and thoughts about the encounters. Facilitators need to model openness to varying perceptions of workplace aggressions and foster discussion in ways that do not impede participation. Learning activities are provided to promote meaningful discussion on these sensitive topics. However, bear in mind that some learners may withdraw and offer little or nothing to the conversation as a means of self-protection. For example, if a learner has experienced physical violence from a student or patient, they may display a range of emotions and be reticent to discuss the situation since, for some individuals, witnessing or being on the receiving end of workplace aggressions can make a negative and lasting impression. Facilitators can remind learners that they are only asked to share information they are comfortable sharing.

In addition to small and large group discussion sessions, be sure to provide alternate opportunities for learners to share their thoughts such as using anonymous polling apps, formative assessment techniques, clickers, or free-writes that do not include the learner's name or other identifying information. Remember that perception plays a key role in how individuals view behaviors and experiences. For example, what might be considered an act of incivility will vary from individual to individual. Perceptions are influenced by the people involved, the situation, type of relationship, delivery, tone, and context.

Given the sensitive nature and varying perspectives of the content contained in Chapter 2, along with the complexity of facilitating learning activities associated with the material, it may be helpful to incorporate a formative assessment at the end of class. Formative assessments are brief, ungraded, anonymous, end-of-class activities designed to provide facilitators with feedback regarding the quality and effectiveness of the learning activities. Formative assessments also help to identify gaps in learning and provide information about the quality of facilitation and how to plan subsequent learning activities (Oermann et al., 2018). An example of a formative assessment for this chapter follows based on the Critical Incident Questionnaire (CIQ) created by Brookfield (2015), a tool that allows facilitators to "see the classroom through students' eyes" (p. 34).

CIQ in the Classroom

At the end of class, the facilitator distributes the formative assessment (or CIQ) either in hard copy or online. The assessment is completed anonymously, and if nothing comes to mind as a response to a particular question, learners can leave the question blank. The CIQ takes three to five minutes to complete. If desired, responses to the CIQ can be summarized, aggregated, and shared with learners during the next class meeting. Here are the five questions:

1. At what moment were you most engaged as a learner?
2. What moment were you most distanced as a learner?
3. What action was taken that was most helpful to your learning?
4. What action was taken that was most puzzling to you?
5. What surprised you most about today's session?

Chapter 2 CIQ Practice

For facilitators interested in assessing learning and application to practice, the following formative assessment may be administered using a process like the CIQ described above:

1. What is the most significant concept, issue, or topic you learned today?
2. What is the one concept, issue, or topic you still need more time to learn?
3. How will this learning experience affect your clinical practice?

While the use of formative assessments is introduced in this chapter of the facilitator guide, they may be used periodically throughout the curriculum. Instead of relying on your own observations as a facilitator, learning activities and teaching techniques are based on feedback coming from the participants themselves.

Key Concepts

After reading the chapter, ask the learners to test their understanding of the concepts with short answers.

1. What are potential risks of experiencing incivility in the workplace for patients?

    Answer: Dissatisfaction with patient experience; dissatisfaction with care quality or not as likely to seek care again in the same facility; greater risk of physical harm; near misses, life-threatening mistakes, preventable complications, or death of a patient.

2. What are potential risks of workplace aggression for healthcare workers?

   Answer: Higher levels of staff disengagement, absenteeism, and turnover. There is a potential for decreased communication about safety concerns and an increased risk of medical errors. Nurses can experience chronic stress from bullying, which can impact their ability to provide safe patient care. Workplace aggressions erode psychological safety and mutual trust among team members. When trust in team members is lost, open communication about safety concerns ceases, medical errors increase, and the ability for an organization to learn from mistakes to prevent recurrent errors is severely impaired.

3. What are potential risks of workplace aggression for nursing educators and students?

   Answer: Incivility in nursing education has harmful physical and psychological effects on both faculty and students and disturbs the teaching-learning environment. Incivility in nursing education can influence unsafe behavior of future nurses in the practice environment, which can negatively impact patient safety.

4. What is the potential impact of workplace aggression on a new nurse's well-being?

   Answer: Evidence from the literature (Laschinger and Read, 2016) suggests that graduate nurses who experienced incivility reported lower career satisfaction and greater intent to leave. New graduate nurses who observed incivility reported negative effects on their emotional, professional, and physical well-being and expressed how uncivil acts in the patient care environment negatively impacted patient safety.

5. What is the Continuum of Workplace Aggression?

   Answer: The Continuum of Workplace Aggression illustrates a progression of how lower-level aggression can escalate into higher-level aggression if unaddressed. Behaviors within the continuum include incivility, microaggressions, bullying, intimidation, mobbing, physical violence, and tragedy.

6. What are the National Institute for Occupational Safety & Health (NIOSH) definitions of violence?

   Answer: According to NIOSH (Centers for Disease Control & Prevention, 2020), workplace violence includes direct physical assaults, written or verbal threats, physical or verbal harassment, and homicide. NIOSH has identified four types of workplace violence in the healthcare field: Type I involves criminal intent; type II involves a customer, client, or patient; type III involves worker-on-worker violence; and type IV involves personal relationships.

7. Why don't nurses report workplace aggression?

   Answer: Evidence from a recent national study (Clark et al., 2021) found that academic nurse leaders and faculty avoided dealing with incivility for several reasons, including fear of retaliation, lack of supervisor or administrator support, and the fact that addressing incivility can make matters worse.

Rationale for Implementation

After reading the chapter, ask the learners to test their understanding of the concepts with short answers.

1. Why is it important for nurses, healthcare providers, and educators to identify and understand the impact of workplace aggression?

    Answer: Workplace aggression occurs on a continuum, and low-level behaviors such as uncivil nonverbal behaviors and sarcasm need to be identified and addressed to prevent such behaviors from escalating into more aggressive behaviors such as intimidation, threats, physical violence, or tragedy.

2. Why is it important to report workplace aggression?

    Answer: Unreported workplace aggression can contribute to unsafe patient care, poor outcomes for healthcare workers, and a culture of incivility.

Application of the Concepts

Working in pairs and individually, instruct learners to complete the following exercises.

1. Paired Activity: Sharing an Uncivil Encounter

The following is a think-pair-share activity that integrates a narrative pedagogy approach. If in a larger group, ask learners to pair up and go through the following activity with one another (provide in-session time to complete the activity), and then have them share their biggest takeaway points to the larger group.

Recall an uncivil encounter you had in the past in nursing, healthcare, or the education setting. Think about the events preceding it, the event, and the aftermath. Then, share this experience and reflections about it in a conversation with a trusted friend or colleague. Ask your colleague to share their thoughts on the following questions regarding the event.

1. Have you ever experienced something like this?
2. How would you feel if you experienced this situation?
3. If faced with this situation, what would you do? Explain your reasoning.

Once finished, learners may switch with the friend or colleague and ask them to share their experience, and they can share their responses to the same set of questions.

Pairs are asked to share their biggest takeaways from their discussions with the larger group.

2. Case Narrative Activity: Bystander of an Uncivil Shift Report

The following is a problem-based learning activity for a group discussion. Explain that this narrative represents a real-life situation, and ask learners to consider the situation as if it were occurring in real time. Give learners 10 to 15 minutes to read the following narrative, reflect on the content and impact of the situation, and respond to the questions that follow by taking notes. Then, the facilitator leads a discussion using the narrative and the discussion questions that follow.

Narrative: The Case of the Bystander of an Uncivil Shift Report

Lindsey, a staff registered nurse, enters a busy oncology unit at the beginning of her shift and witnesses a heated, uncivil exchange from an oncoming nurse who is already receiving report from an off-going nurse. The situation is about tasks left undone, and the oncoming nurse is angry and talking down to the nurse who was giving report and soon to be off shift: "You've got to be kidding me. Really? What have you done all shift? Why can't you manage your time better? I'm sick and tired of cleaning up after you!" The off-going nurse appears intimidated and shocked at what is happening.

Questions:

1. If you were the third-party nurse witnessing the event, how would you feel?
2. What would you do or not do, and why?
3. How might this situation impact the clinical setting and patient care?
4. What are some barriers to addressing the situation?
5. What measures might you take to overcome these barriers?

Reflection

The process of reflection helps learners become more self-aware, problem-solve, and identify motivators and barriers that may impact how they recognize and address challenging situations. Learners can engage in reflective practice through dialogue in small and large groups, writing activities such as journaling or free-writes, or scriptwriting and storytelling. Facilitators can encourage learners to use one or more of these reflective practices to respond to the following questions.

1. Did your perspective about the impact of workplace aggression change after reading this chapter? Why or why not? If it did change, describe what you learned and how it informs your future practice.

2. Let's say you witnessed low-level uncivil behavior in the workplace since having read this chapter. What are the potential implications of leaving this behavior unaddressed? How motivated would you be to address uncivil behavior, knowing the impact it can have on patient safety? What would be a barrier to addressing uncivil behavior as a witness, and how could you overcome this barrier?

Objective: Learners share personal reflections and perceptions of their experiences related to workplace aggressions and their impacts.

References

Brookfield, S. (2015). *The skillful teacher: On technique, trust, and responsiveness in the classroom.* Jossey-Bass.

Centers for Disease Control and Prevention. (2020, September 22). National Institute for Occupational Safety and Health (NIOSH). *Occupational violence.* https://www.cdc.gov/niosh/topics/violence/default.html

Clark, C. M., Landis, T., & Barbosa-Leiker, C. (2021). National study on faculty and administrators' perceptions of civility and incivility in nursing education. *Nurse Educator, 46*(5), 276–283. doi: 10.1097/NNE.0000000000000948

Laschinger, H. K., & Read, E. A. (2016). The effect of authentic leadership, person-job fit, and civility norms on new graduate nurses' experiences of coworker incivility and burnout. *Journal of Nursing Administration, 46*(11), 574–580. https://doi.org/10.1097/nna.0000000000000407

Oermann, M. H., DeGagne, J. C., & Phillips, B. C. (2018). *Teaching in nursing and the role of the educator: The complete guide to best practices in teaching, evaluation, and curriculum development* (2nd ed.). Springer Publishing.

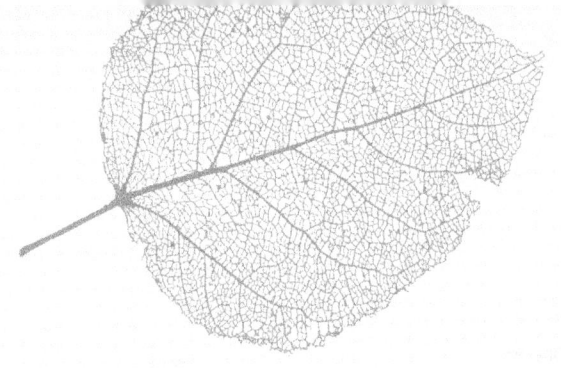

3

The Power and Imperative of Self-Awareness

LEARNING OUTCOMES

- Define emotional intelligence and its relationship to self-awareness.
- Explain the importance of self-awareness for fostering civil relationships.
- Describe at least two strategies to improve self-awareness.
- Discuss how explicit and implicit biases might contribute to incivility.
- Utilize the IAT from Project Implicit to increase self-awareness about potential implicit biases.

Before You Begin

Chapter 3 emphasizes the importance of self-awareness as a component of developing and honing emotional intelligence. To be self-aware is to know ourselves as we really are and realize that this process is a lifelong journey as we peel back the layers of our identity to reveal our true essence (Bradberry & Greaves, 2009). Enhancing emotional intelligence and deepening self-awareness are key components to becoming a more skilled facilitator, developing positive relationships with learners, thriving in the educator role, and building personal resilience. Being self-aware and, in turn, helping learners become more self-aware means understanding how emotions and thoughts influence behavior and how making accurate (or inaccurate) assessments of our strengths and limitations impacts others, and how their behavior impacts us. In other words, self-awareness means seeing ourselves clearly and objectively, understanding our emotions and the effect on self and others, knowing what we feel and why, and recognizing how we are perceived by others.

As facilitators, we bring ourselves to the learning environment. Emotions and experiences can influence how we conduct class and respond to learners. Discussing uncivil encounters and other workplace aggressions can create anxiety in learners, activate unpleasant emotions, and uncover unresolved issues in their lives—as well as the facilitator's life. Therefore, it is important for facilitators to be aware of their emotional triggers and manage them in a poised and professional manner, in such a way as to avoid power struggles. Facilitators are encouraged to develop effective strategies for self-awareness before facilitating content on this topic.

One way to enhance self-awareness is to uncover and deconstruct the issues or behaviors that push our buttons. What are your pet peeves, triggers, or hot buttons that annoy you, irritate you, or make you feel uncomfortable? Jot them down in a journal and explore the sources of these hot buttons. Then, make a list of strategies to lessen the impact of your hot buttons and practice implementing them before class. Knowing what pushes your buttons and developing the ability to take control of these situations is evidence of a skilled and experienced facilitator.

In Chapter 3, the Workplace Civility Index© and the Everyday Civility Index© are provided to assess civility acumen at work and in everyday life. Facilitators may also wish to avail themselves of the Faculty Civility Index© to assess civility within the educator role (Clark, 2017).

Some of the items on the Faculty Civility Index include asking yourself, do I:

- Regard students as adult learners and expect them to succeed?
- Role-model civility, professionalism, and respectful discourse?
- Believe learners add value and meaning to the educational experience?
- Come to class prepared and use evidence-based teaching/learning strategies?

- Listen to and incorporate constructive feedback into my teaching practices?
- Demonstrate an openness to other points of view?
- Include, welcome, encourage, and mentor learners?

Facilitators might also ask themselves:

- What would it be like to be on the receiving end of me?
- How do I respond when my buttons are pushed?
- In the best of all worlds, how would I like to respond when my buttons are pushed?

Encouraging learners to enhance their level of self-awareness is disingenuous if facilitators have not engaged in similar exercises and activities. Consider implementing some of the strategies designed to assess and mitigate bias (both conscious and unconscious) provided in Chapter 3. Challenge yourself to complete at least one of the Implicit Association Tests (IAT) provided by Project Implicit (2011).

Sharing your insights with a trusted colleague before facilitating class and being mindful of how your actions and emotions affect others as well as the learning environment can help reduce the potential of bringing personal biases into the classroom. Developing facilitation skills requires open, honest self-reflection and being willing to incorporate helpful feedback from trusted colleagues on ways to improve your teaching expertise.

In the words of Parker Palmer (2017), "We can speak to the teacher within our students only when we are on speaking terms with the teacher within ourselves" (p. 32). In other words, when teaching or facilitating comes from the depths of our own truth and self-awareness, the truth and awareness within students have a chance to respond in kind.

Key Concepts

After reading the chapter, ask the learners to test their understanding of the concepts with short answers.

1. How would you define emotional intelligence?

    Answer: *Emotional intelligence* refers to the ability of a person to perceive, generate, and regulate emotions to promote emotional and intellectual growth for oneself as well as in relationships with others.

2. What is the relationship between emotional intelligence and self-awareness?

    Answer: According to Goleman (1995), the five competencies of emotional intelligence are: self-regulation, motivation, empathy, social skills, and self-awareness. While all five competencies are essential for enhancing emotional intelligence, *self-awareness* is highlighted in this chapter. Self-awareness is the ability to understand our emotions, strengths, areas for improvement, and drives—and realize and appreciate their effect upon self and others.

3. Identify at least two strategies to improve self-awareness.

    Answer: Several strategies are presented by the author, such as self-reflection exercises including the Workplace Civility Index (WCI), the Everyday Civility Index (ECI), and asking for or incorporating feedback from trusted colleagues, friends, or family members (Clark, 2017). In addition, learners can ask themselves probing questions to enhance their self-awareness. There are tools and instruments to uncover implicit biases, such as using the Implicit Association Test (IAT) through Project Implicit.

4. Define explicit and implicit bias.

    Answer: *Explicit bias* refers to holding conscious attitudes and beliefs about a person or group. In contrast, *implicit bias* is an unconscious, negative set of attitudes and beliefs about a group and its members in comparison to another group.

5. How do explicit and implicit biases relate to incivility?

    Answer: Expressing explicit biases against groups and individuals could influence uncivil behaviors toward others. Implicit bias is also concerning because it could influence uncivil behavior on an unconscious level, which is more difficult for people to mitigate because it is not readily recognized but still exists and could pose harm to others.

Rationale for Implementation

After reading the chapter, ask the learners to test their understanding of the concepts with short answers.

1. Why is improving self-awareness important to fostering civil relationships?

    Answer: Practicing self-awareness activities helps people reflect, acknowledge, and understand their triggers, hot buttons, and patterns of behavior that could impact others in the workplace, which is critical to modifying behaviors as needed to promote civil relationships.

2. Why is it important to acknowledge explicit and implicit biases in relation to civility in nursing and healthcare?

    Answer: Acknowledging explicit and implicit biases is a critical first step to replacing thoughts of stereotypic judgment with non-biased thoughts, which might help improve health outcomes for vulnerable minority patient groups.

Application of the Concepts

Working in small groups and with a partner, instruct learners to complete the following exercises.

1. Group Activity: Using the Implicit Association Test to Build Self-Awareness

If possible, have learners complete at least one Implicit Association Test (IAT) provided by Project Implicit on their device prior to the learning activity (https://implicit.harvard.edu/implicit/). If completing the IAT before class is not feasible, provide class time for learners to complete the assignment. This IAT self-awareness activity incorporates reflection and small group discussion. After completing the IAT activity, ask learners to gather in small groups and share their biggest takeaway points. This could include how they were impacted by what they learned and how it will affect their behavior in the future. If time permits, a spokesperson from each small group can share lessons learned with the larger group.

In small groups, ask learners to share their insights to the following questions:

1. Which IAT did you complete? What factors motivated you to select this test?
2. Using only one word, how would you describe the IAT experience?
3. Which results or findings from the IAT surprised you the most?
4. Which results or findings from the IAT concerned you the most?
5. What action(s) would you take based on the findings from your IAT?

2. Paired Activity: Understanding the Impact of Biased Statements

Provide class time for learners to pair up and take turns reading the biased statements listed below aloud to one another. Each pair can take turns answering the following seven questions and discuss major takeaway points from the experience. One person from each pair can then share their lessons learned, or major takeaway points, with the larger group.

Listed below are examples of biased statements that may be considered uncivil.

- "Old people are boring."
- "This patient is a frequent flyer."
- "People from small towns are uneducated."
- "Asians are great at math."
- "Most male nurses are gay."
- "All adolescents are addicted to social media."
- "Overweight people are lazy."

Ask learners to discuss the following questions:

1. After reading the examples aloud, what effect did they have on you?
2. Have you been on the receiving end, or observed, biased statements?
3. How did experiencing or witnessing biased statements impact you?
4. If you have witnessed or experienced statements like these in the workplace, how did you respond or not respond?
5. If you chose to respond, what was the outcome?
6. If you chose not to respond, what was the outcome?
7. What might you do differently in the future?

Ask learners to volunteer some of their responses with the class.

Reflection

The process of reflection helps learners become more self-aware, introspective, and mindful of the impact their behaviors have on others and the work environment. Reflective activities provide an opportunity for inquiry and a mechanism for questioning ideas, assumptions, and beliefs. When learners share their insights and perspectives with others, it provides an opportunity to receive feedback and additional points of view from other individuals.

For this reflection exercise, learners can choose to complete the Workplace Civility Index or the Everyday Civility Index provided in Chapter 3.

To complete the index of choice, have learners find a quiet place, free from distractions, and honestly assess their level of civility. Then, have them respond to the following questions:

1. How satisfied are you with your overall civility score?
2. Are there examples of civility where you excel?
3. Are there examples of civility you wish to improve? Briefly describe them.
4. In the most honest way possible, determine one or more areas for civility improvement and personal growth. Then identify one or more strategies you will implement to improve an area of civility and personal growth. Include your proposed timeline for implementation.
5. In the most honest way possible, identify one or more areas of strength. Then identify one or more strategies you will implement to continue developing these strengths. Include your proposed timeline for implementation.

Once learners have completed their index of choice and responded to these questions, have them select a classmate, colleague, or friend and take turns sharing their insights and reflections.

Objective: Learners share personal reflections and perceptions of their experiences related to personal civility, incivility, and strategies for change.

References

Bradberry, T., & Greaves, J. (2009). *Emotional intelligence 2.0*. TalentSmart.

Clark, C. M. (2017). *Creating and sustaining civility in nursing education* (2nd ed.). Sigma Theta Tau International.

Goleman, D. (1995). *Emotional intelligence: Why it can matter more than IQ*. Bantam.

Palmer, P. J. (2017). *The courage to teach: Exploring the inner landscape of a teacher's life*. Jossey-Bass.

Project Implicit. (2011). *Implicit Association Test*. https://implicit.harvard.edu/implicit/

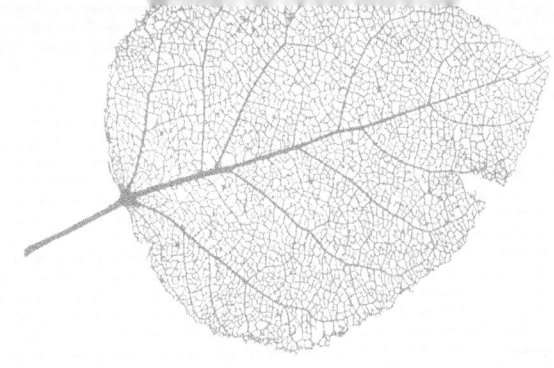

4

Practicing the Fundamentals of Civility

LEARNING OUTCOMES

- Define what it means to be a civilist.
- Explain how expressing gratitude is a fundamental element of civility.
- Describe how living by the Platinum Rule is a fundamental element of civility.
- Define how conveying empathy is a fundamental element of civility.
- Explain how listening well is a fundamental element of civility.
- Describe how expressing micro-affirmations is a fundamental element of civility.

Before You Begin

Chapter 4 focuses on the fundamentals of becoming a civilist and a role model for professionalism, civility, and respectful interactions. Fundamentals are the most basic, uncomplicated, key features of a concept or construct. Practicing and honing the fundamentals of civility includes expressing gratitude, living by the Platinum Rule, conveying empathy, listening well, and expressing micro-affirmations. To perform these functions well, it's important to intentionally notice how we behave and interact with others during everyday interactions. As with any subject, identifying, understanding, and practicing the fundamentals of civility are important to developing individual and organizational competencies of civility, protecting worker and patient safety, and fostering healthy work environments. Fundamentals are critical, yet rarely discussed and reinforced because people assume everyone understands them.

To illustrate, consider fundamentals within the context of athletics. Successful coaches explain, clarify, and demonstrate the fundamentals of their sport. They provide players with ample opportunities to practice and receive feedback on the execution of the game's fundamentals. If players fail to practice and hone the fundamentals of their sport, they will have difficulty performing on game day. The same concept can be applied to nursing and healthcare. When teaching the essential elements or principles of civility, facilitators must stress the fundamentals so that learners can be successful in the workplace. When nurses and other healthcare professionals practice and master the fundamentals of civility, they are better equipped to prevent and address uncivil situations and protect the safety and well-being of self and others.

When the fundamentals of civility are neglected, patient outcomes are suboptimal, and uncivil situations may lead to serious consequences. On the other hand, when fundamental skills are improved and consistently practiced over time, they become more instinctive and natural. Addressing the basics of civility may be accomplished through reflective practices, which can be achieved by creating a safe, positive learning environment and fostering a trusting relationship between facilitators and learners (Barbagallo, 2021; Bjerkvik & Hilli, 2019).

Throughout our professional lives, improving the fundamental skills of civility will prove to be invaluable. Chapter 4 highlights five civility fundamentals: 1) expressing gratitude, 2) living by the Platinum Rule, 3) conveying empathy, 4) listening well, and 5) expressing micro-affirmations. Facilitating meaningful discussions about these concepts with learners requires facilitators to reflect on their own behaviors and take careful inventory on how they do or do not model the civility fundamentals. For example, facilitators should model empathy, welcome and value other points of view, strive to see the world through the eyes of others, and practice perspective-taking.

Extending appreciation for learner contributions is also important. Facilitators can express appreciation and recognition by commending learners for their input, effort, enthusiasm, and application of the course material. Brookfield (2015) notes that showing appreciation for learner contributions is one of the most neglected behaviors in education and suggests using an appreciative pause to build cohesion in a group dealing with sensitive issues. To use an appreciative pause, at least once during each discussion, the facilitator calls for a one-minute pause. During this time, the only comments allowed from learners are those that acknowledge how something that someone said in the discussion (not the facilitator) has contributed to their learning. This can lead to listening well, paying attention, and genuinely valuing what learners offer to the class discussion. Following the Platinum Rule by doing unto others as they would want done unto them can be reinforced in the classroom. Sharing micro-affirmations in the classroom might include giving credit to learners, providing support, and affirming the contributions of others. These skills can be improved with supportive effort, guidance, and meaningful facilitation.

Key Concepts

After reading the chapter, ask the learners to test their understanding of the concepts with short answers.

1. Define and describe the characteristics of a civilist.

    Answer: A civilist is someone who consistently models the attributes and qualities of a respectful person, honors and advocates for diversity and inclusivity, exhibits principled character, demonstrates responsible citizenship, invites and values the perspectives of others, and fosters a genuine sense of belonging. Being a civilist means being recognized as a person who consistently promotes civility in one's personal and professional life.

2. Define and give an example of each of the five fundamentals of civility.

    Answer:

    - **Expressing gratitude** means taking the time to show genuine appreciation, thank others, and recognize others' contributions. One example is nurses thanking colleagues who help them with patient care upon admitting new patients to a hospital unit.

    - **Living by the Platinum Rule** means doing unto others as they would want done unto them. For example, asking a trainee in their first position as a registered nurse the following question is demonstrating thoughtfulness and care of others' desires and needs: "What is the most challenging aspect of orienting to this position as a new nurse, and how can I help you develop in this role?"

    - **Conveying empathy** means communicating to others that you understand their perspective and are able to envision it from their point of view rather than one's own. Empathy can be conveyed by listening to another person's point of view to understand their perspective and communicate appreciation for their opinions or beliefs.

    - **Listening well** means being present and engaged in receiving communication from another person. One example of listening well is putting down other activities and electronic devices and stating, "I'm listening," while actively thinking about what the other is saying.

- **Expressing micro-affirmations** means acknowledging others' contributions in small acts to help others succeed. One example is stating, "Great job! You inspire me to continue doing my best work."

Rationale for Implementation

After reading the chapter, ask the learners to test their understanding of the concepts with short answers.

1. Why is it important to strive to be a civilist according to the author's definition?

   Answer: Practicing and mastering the fundamentals of civility can help nurses and other healthcare professionals prevent and address uncivil situations. Becoming a civilist helps to protect the safety and well-being of self and others.

2. Why is it important to identify, understand, and practice the fundamentals of civility in nursing and healthcare?

   Answer: As with any subject, identifying, understanding, and practicing the fundamentals or the key elements of civility are important to developing individual and organizational competencies of civility, protecting patient and worker safety, and fostering healthy work environments.

Application of the Concepts

Working in small groups and independently, instruct learners to complete the following exercises.

1. Group Activity: Reflection on What It Means to Be a Civilist

The following activity is a reflective practice exercise that combines action and reflection. Active reflection on learning outcomes and key concepts transforms the learner from a passive recipient of someone else's thoughts to an active constructor of knowledge and meaning (Oermann et al., 2018). This activity provides a rich opportunity for learners to analyze the author's definition of a new concept and construct additional meaning with an emphasis on application to practice.

To begin, provide time for each learner to work independently to respond to the following questions. Following this independent exercise, have learners assemble into small groups of five to six participants. Provide time for learners to share their responses with the group. Encourage dialogue and feedback among the participants.

1. For many learners, the term *civilist* may be a new concept. After reflecting on the author's definition of a civilist, consider how this concept resonates with you in your nursing or healthcare role.

2. Does the author's characterization align with your definition of a civilist? If not, how might you amend the definition?

3. As you consider your role in nursing or healthcare:

- Which aspects of the civilist definition apply to you most?

- Which aspects of the civilist definition apply to you least?

- How will you implement the elements of your civilist definition into your nursing or healthcare practice and/or learning environment?

2. Free-Write Activity: Applying the Fundamentals of Civility

Have learners bring their laptop, tablet, or smartphone to class. This learning exercise combines an internet search with a free-write activity. First, have learners conduct a search of the five fundamentals of civility discussed in Chapter 4: 1) expressing gratitude, 2) living by the Platinum Rule, 3) conveying empathy, 4) listening well, and 5) expressing micro-affirmations. Have students take notes on the results of their search and identify one civility fundamental that resonates or intrigues them the most. Once the search is completed, use a 10-minute free-write activity to have learners respond to the following questions. If time permits, have learners share a key takeaway with the large group.

Free-writes are an excellent way to cultivate thinking and construct ideas. Grammar, spelling, and punctuation do not matter. Using pen and paper or a keyboard, the goal is to express ideas and thoughts about a specific topic within an allotted time frame. Free-writes serve as an effective warmup exercise for class discussion and help get the cognitive and affective juices flowing (Clark, 2017). As a rule, free-writes are not formally graded; instead, facilitators can use them to generate conversation and seek deeper understanding of the concepts. Freewriting allows learners to express ideas in an open and unrestricted manner that might not otherwise surface through more conventional means.

1. After conducting an internet search on the five fundamentals of civility, select one fundamental that resonates or intrigues you the most.

2. During a 10-minute free-write, describe how you would integrate this fundamental concept into your work or learning environment.

Reflection

To become a civilist, it is important to reflect on behavior that is, and is not, consistent with being a respectful person, and to think about strategies to consistently demonstrate respect. To improve civility acumen, ask learners to reflect on a time when they or someone they know was treated in a disrespectful or demeaning manner. Then, ask them to share their answers to the following questions with a trusted colleague, friend, or family member.

1. Briefly describe the uncivil or disrespectful situation or encounter.

2. As you witnessed or experienced the situation or encounter:
    - What feelings were evoked?
    - How did you respond to the situation or encounter?
    - Were other individuals involved in the situation or encounter? If so, how did they respond?

Now, ask learners to think of a time when they were affirmed and made to feel valued and respected—their efforts celebrated.

1. Briefly describe the experience of being affirmed and valued by others.

2. As you experienced being affirmed and valued by others:
    - What feelings were evoked?
    - How did you respond to the affirmation?
    - Were there other individuals involved in the experience? If so, how did they respond?

Have learners reflect on opportunities to integrate micro-affirmations in their everyday work, such as during team meetings or through personal communication. Have them create a list of micro-affirmations that they can use in their work setting and in everyday encounters.

To help them get started, refer to these examples from page 65 of the book:

- You are absolutely one of the best problem-solvers I know. Thanks!
- You have really opened my eyes and helped me see things in a new light.
- Congratulations on your promotion. It is well deserved.
- Having you on the team has been a game-changer for us.

Facilitator tip: Once learners have created a list of micro-affirmations, have them share their insights with a trusted colleague, friend, or family member.

References

Barbagallo, M. S. (2021). Nursing students' perceptions and experiences of reflective practice: A qualitative meta-synthesis. *Teaching and Learning in Nursing, 16*(1), 24–31. doi: 10.1016/j.teln.2020.07.006

Bjerkvik, L. K., & Hilli, Y. (2019). Reflective writing in undergraduate clinical nursing education: A literature review. *Nurse Education in Practice, 35*, 32–41. doi:10.1016/j.nepr.2018.11.013

Brookfield, S. (2015). *The skillful teacher: On technique, trust, and responsiveness in the classroom.* Jossey-Bass.

Clark, C. M. (2017). *Creating and sustaining civility in nursing education* (2nd ed.). Indianapolis, IN: Sigma Theta Tau International.

Oermann, M. H., DeGagne, J. C., & Phillips, B. C. (2018). *Teaching in nursing and the role of the educator: The complete guide to best practices in teaching, evaluation, and curriculum development* (2nd ed.). Springer Publishing.

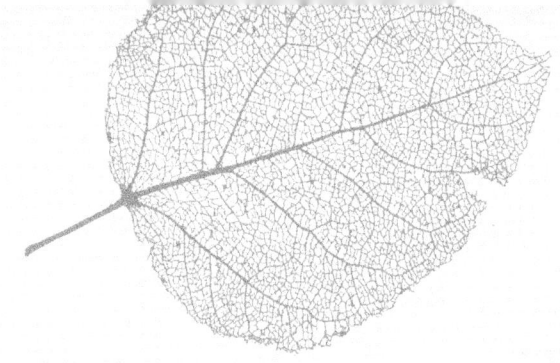

5

Honing Communication Skills and Conflict Competence

LEARNING OUTCOMES

- Understand the meaning of POWER skills.
- Apply the individual conflict-competence model.
- Employ "I" statements effectively.
- Use learning scripts and phrases to address uncivil or conflicted situations.
- Implement evidence-based frameworks to prevent and address incivility and protect worker and patient safety.

Before You Begin

For most people, addressing uncivil behaviors and managing conflict are challenging, often daunting endeavors. Facilitators providing learning activities that touch sensitive topics such as conflict and disagreement—or, as in this chapter, uncivil and bullying encounters—must be aware that learners may be affected by memories of their own experiences with incivility and other aggressive behaviors. Facilitators must have a sound working knowledge of the content of civility and incivility, and, more importantly, respect the impact of incivility and other aggressions on individuals, teams, organizations, and patient care.

The learning activities contained in this chapter include the use of Cognitive Rehearsal (CR), a technique used in behavioral science whereby learners work with a skilled facilitator to discuss and rehearse effective ways to address a problem or social situation. CR is a sophisticated pedagogical technique led by a skilled and experienced facilitator and debriefer. In this chapter, role-play is used within the context of CR and is designed to educate learners on ways to recognize and respond to incivility and other workplace aggressions. Role-play as a teaching-learning technique enables learners to act out various roles within the scenarios, analyze activities and dynamics occurring during the role-play, and share observations and reactions during a structured debriefing session following the activity.

While engaging with incivility content, some learners may experience an array of emotions such as anxiety, tension, apprehension, or other feelings of discomfort. To mitigate the effects of potential unease or distress, some scholars advocate for the use of trigger or content warnings. Content warnings consider the possibility that learners may be triggered (in a psychological sense) by stressful content and provide a simple heads-up about the content to be discussed (Gannon, 2020). The primary intent of a content warning is to help prepare learners as much as possible to constructively engage and interact with the course content and activities. While the use of content warnings remains somewhat controversial with critics on both sides (Gannon, 2020; Palfrey, 2018), those who advocate for the use of content warnings believe they provide the structure and support necessary for genuine dialogue to occur by creating an environment where ideas can receive the engagement they deserve. An example of a content warning for this chapter follows:

Today we will be role-playing scenarios that depict a range of uncivil and other aggressive encounters. The scenarios portray real-life experiences that you may find unsettling or that may remind you of events that happened in your life. If you need to take a short break or speak with me privately after class, please let me know.

As with any experience or event that may produce an undesirable emotional or psychological response, be sure to provide learners with campus, organizational, or community resources to offer support.

Key Concepts

After reading the chapter, ask the learners to test their understanding of the concepts with short answers.

1. What does the author mean by POWER skills?

    Answer: Effective communication and constructive conflict negotiation.

2. Why are POWER skills challenging to master?

    Answer: Correct answers should explain that POWER skills are challenging to master because individuals and situations can be so varied. Every encounter is different—it occurs in a different environment, involves different individuals within different contexts, uses a different tone or delivery, and so on.

3. Why might it be helpful to think of a situation as a "controversy with civility" rather than as a "conflict?"

    Answer: Correct answers should note that "conflict" implies an us vs. them winner/loser mindset, while "controversy with civility" suggests that the parties can negotiate a mutually agreeable solution. The main principles of controversy with civility include 1) differences in viewpoint are inevitable, and 2) differences must be expressed honestly with civility and an openness for opposing points of view.

4. Why is it important for nurses, faculty, students, and others to identify their hot buttons and to implement strategies to mitigate the effects of these hot buttons?

    Answer: Hot buttons are behaviors displayed by others that tend to trigger negative emotions and strong reactions that lead to the use of destructive behaviors. Being aware of hot buttons helps an individual develop action plans to address conflict in a more constructive manner.

5. What are the three steps of the individual conflict competence model?

    Answer:

    a. Cool down

    b. Slow down and reflect

    c. Engage constructively

6. Based on the work of Maxfield and Grenny (2017), describe two common reasons why a nurse might fail to speak up, even though patient safety is at stake.

    Answer: There are five main categories of possible correct responses: unmotivated peers, difficult peers, poor leadership, favoritism, and unresponsive physicians.

7. List the five steps for using "I" statements effectively.

   Answer:

   Step 1: Listen for understanding.

   Step 2: Use "I" statements to express your point of view.

   Step 3: Refer to the behavior and not the person.

   Step 4: State how the behavior affects you or makes you feel.

   Step 5: State what you would like to happen.

8. What are some benefits of using "I" statements when communicating and or attempting to resolve conflict?

   Answer: Correct answers should include at least two of the following benefits: help clarify our position, assist in preserving or improving relationships rather than making them worse, and help get the conversation started and moving forward in a constructive manner.

9. List the six steps of the Caring Feedback Model.

   Answer:

   Step 1. State positive intent/purpose.

   Step 2. Ask permission to give feedback.

   Step 3. Describe the specific behavior.

   Step 4. Explain the consequence/impact (for you, your team, your patients/students, or the organization).

   Step 5. Offer a pinch of empathy.

   Step 6. Make a suggestion or request.

10. List the three considerations of the CUS Model.

    Answer:

    Step 1: I am **c**oncerned.

    Step 2: I am **u**ncomfortable.

    Step 3: This is a **s**afety issue.

11. List the four steps of the DESC Model.

    Answer:

    Step 1: **D**escribe the situation or behavior.

    Step 2: **E**xpress your concerns about the situation.

Step 3: **S**uggest alternatives and seek agreement.

Step 4: **C**onsequences stated while striving for consensus.

12. List the five steps of the PAAIL Method.

    Answer:

    Step 1: **P**review: I'd like to talk to you about _____.

    Step 2: **A**dvocacy (Part 1): I saw (or heard or noticed) _____.

    Step 3: **A**dvocacy (Part 2): I am concerned because _____.

    Step 4: **I**nquiry: I wonder what was on your mind at the time?

    Step 5: **L**isten: Listen carefully and intentionally to response.

Rationale for Implementation

After reading the chapter, ask the learners to test their understanding of the concepts with short answers.

1. In what ways can strong POWER skills improve patient care, learner engagement, and workplace civility?

   Answer: Points of discussion that should be covered are that they lead to better outcomes, improve collaboration and teamwork, and ultimately protect worker and patient safety.

2. What are some characteristics of a good listener? Do you have a good listener in your life? Share an example with a colleague, friend, or classmate.

   Answer: The goal of this discussion question is to draw learners out to share examples and help each other note the common characteristics described.

Application of the Concepts

When teaching this material, the author likes to use a technique called Cognitive Rehearsal (CR), a behavioral strategy whereby groups and individuals work with a skilled facilitator to practice and rehearse effective ways to address uncivil encounters. Facilitators of CR use role-play and simulation to have individuals repeatedly rehearse an uncivil situation, while simultaneously coaching the person to use effective communication and conflict skills and then debriefing the situation (Clark, 2019; Clark & Gorton, 2019; Griffin, 2004; Griffin & Clark, 2014;). This is a powerful combination of skill sets and is more likely to lead to a successful outcome, improve collaboration and teamwork, and ultimately protect worker and patient safety.

Working in pairs and with a small group, instruct learners to complete the following exercises.

1. Paired Activity: Using "I" Statements Effectively

Pair up learners and direct them to review the five steps of using "I" statements. Using the following narrative, the pair should play the roles and practice using "I" statements to resolve the conflict. Then they should switch roles and practice them again.

Narrative: The Case of Intrusive Behavior From a Colleague

Professor Chan is an established, tenured faculty member recently hired at a new university. Professor Chan does not share a lot about herself or about her other teaching and service duties outside of research, but her focus on an established program of research is public. Professor Kelley, a practice and teaching expert colleague and longtime employee of the institution, stops Professor Chan in the hallway of their office and begins to ask pointed and personal questions about her workload and responsibilities. Professor Kelley asked a particularly loaded question, which was, "What do you do with all of your time if you aren't teaching?" Later, Professor Chan overhears Professor Kelley discussing Professor Chan with another colleague in the building, stating, "Everyone here teaches; it's what we are known for in this department. The other faculty work hard teaching the students, going to clinical sites, and grading. Why does Professor Chan get special treatment? What does she even do with research?" Professor Chan is concerned that these messages spreading across the department could result in difficulties collaborating with others and decides it is time to address Professor Kelley's concerns in a meeting. Professor Chan is going to use "I" messaging to frame the discussion.

Example of using "I" Statements

"Thank you for meeting with me, Professor Kelley. I wanted to discuss our recent conversation in the hallway. From the conversation, I feel as though the contributions I make through research in the department are being questioned and that I am not doing equal work in the department compared to others. Did I interpret the conversation correctly? I'd like to hear your thoughts, as it would help me better understand your perspective."

Objectives: Becoming familiar with the five steps and using "I" statements effectively. Sometimes learners have difficulty playing one of the roles. Consider providing some time for the pair to write down a script for their roles before actually performing the exercise. Follow up with a discussion of what was most challenging and most comfortable.

2. Paired Activity: Caspersen's Framework

Pair up learners and direct them to use Caspersen's Framework to address the scenario "in the moment" (Casperson, 2014). The pair should take turns playing each role, using the framework: When (the triggering event) happened, I (felt or I believed) ____ because my (need/interest) is important to me. Would you be willing to (request a doable) action?

Narrative: The Case of the Scholar's Uncivil Behavior

Professor Blue is a brilliant scholar but a poor communicator. She often works from home, and when she comes to campus, her door is closed and she rarely interacts with others. Most of the time, this does not pose a problem, but when Professor Grey attempts to talk with Professor Blue about a research project on which they are collaborating, she is consistently unavailable. Professor Grey has tried repeatedly to make an appointment with Professor Blue, but she is not responding to calls, texts, or email messages. The research project is grant-funded, and the quarterly report is due. Finally, Professor Grey receives a return email from Professor Blue and is astonished to discover that the email is copied to the Dean and Director chastising Professor Grey and accusing her of sending harassing messages.

Example of Using Caspersen's Framework

"Good morning, Professor Blue, I appreciate the opportunity to meet with you. When you copied the Dean and Director on an email about our research project, I felt both surprised and betrayed. Our working relationship and the success of our research project is very important to me. Would you be willing to formulate a plan to complete the project on time so that we both have input into the process?"

Objectives: Becoming familiar with Casperson's Framework to be able to effectively intervene. Sometimes learners have difficulty identifying a need/interest or doable action. Follow up with a discussion of what was most challenging and most comfortable.

3. Paired Activity: The Caring Feedback Model

Pair up learners and direct them to review the six steps of the Caring Feedback Model (Language of Caring, n.d.). Using the following narrative, the pair should play the roles and practice using the model to resolve the conflict. Then they should switch roles and practice them again.

Narrative: The Case of the Physician's Rude Behavior Pattern

Susan is the nurse manager of a bustling ICU and strives to foster excellent patient care among the members of her team. Dr. Nu is an experienced hospitalist with a reputation for being impatient with nurses, especially those newly hired or from the float pool. The unit is understaffed and extremely busy, so Julie, a registered nurse, has floated to the unit to help. Julie calls Dr. Nu about a patient concern. Dr. Nu interrupts, laughs, and says, "Is that all you called about? Is this a real nurse?" before listening further to understand the patient condition. Julie restates her concern, and once Dr. Nu understands, he orders the appropriate actions. Julie carries out the orders, and the patient situation improves. However, the exchange between Dr. Nu still troubled Julie. Later in the shift, Julie consults her charge nurse about the matter, who confirms that this is a pattern of behavior that other nurses on the unit tend to tolerate because Dr. Nu is respected for his excellent patient care. Julie decides to speak to the unit nurse manager, Susan, about Dr. Nu's behavior pattern and how it is harmful even though it has become an accepted practice. Susan agrees and decides to respond to Dr. Nu's behavior pattern using the Caring Feedback Model.

Example of Using the Caring Feedback Model

1. State positive intent/purpose: "Dr. Nu, I have deep respect for your expertise in the field of medicine and your excellent patient care."

2. As permission to give feedback: "May I offer an observation?"

3. Describe specific behavior: "I have received feedback from several different nurses that when they call you about a patient, they feel their concerns are dismissed before given full attention."

4. Name the consequence/impact: "This could deter nurses from reaching out to you when patient problems arise that need your attention."

5. Offer a pinch of empathy: "I understand that sometimes it can be frustrating to get a report on the phone and not see the full situation."

6. Make a suggestion or request: "Still, when nurses call, it does not help the patient if the nurse feels their observations are dismissed. Can we brainstorm ways to improve communication so that patient needs are appropriately addressed?"

Objectives: Becoming familiar with the Caring Feedback Model to be able to effectively resolve conflict. Sometimes learners have difficulty identifying a point of empathy or determining the suggestion/request. Follow up with a discussion of what was most challenging and most comfortable.

4. Paired Activity: Concerned, Uncomfortable, and Safety (CUS) Model

Pair up learners and direct them to review the three steps of the CUS Model from TeamSTEPPS® 2.0 (Agency for Healthcare Research and Quality, 2021). Using the following narrative, the pair should play the roles and practice using the model to resolve the conflict. Then they should switch roles and practice them again.

Narrative: The Case of the Off-Going Nurse's Uncivil Handoff

Terry is a registered nurse who works at a busy cardiac unit at a large urban regional hospital. She cares for her mother living with Alzheimer's disease and has been experiencing difficulties arriving to places on time due to her role as a caretaker. She was late that morning to her shift at the cardiac unit, and Tia, the off-going nurse, provided her with the following handoff: "Geez, Terry, where have you been? You're late as usual. It's been a crazy, busy shift and I can't wait to get out of here. See if you can manage to get this information straight for once. You should know the patient in 204—you took care of her yesterday, so you should know what's going on. She was on 4S forever. Now she is our problem. She has a bunch of treatments that need to be done and medications that need to be given. You need to check her vital signs too—I've been way too busy to do them. So, that's it—I'm out of here. If I forgot something, it's not my problem. Just check the record."

Example of Using the CUS Model

"Tia, I realize being late is not OK, and we can talk about that later. For now, I'm concerned about Mrs. Tolly and am uncomfortable rushing through your report. For her safety, please provide a complete report before you go."

Objectives: Becoming familiar with the CUS Model to be able to intervene quickly when patient safety is at risk. Follow up with a discussion of what was most challenging and most comfortable.

5. Paired Activity: DESC Model

Pair up learners and direct them to review the four steps of the DESC Model from TeamSTEPPS® 2.0 (AHRQ, 2021). Using the following narrative, the pair should play the roles and practice using the model to resolve the conflict. Then they should switch roles and practice them again.

Narrative: The Case of Co-Teaching in Nursing Education

Professor Brown, DNP, RN, is a part-time clinical lecturer in a college of nursing. She wears many hats both inside the college as a clinical lecturer and outside the college, as she is also a family nurse practitioner with a thriving practice. Professor Brown likes to keep on the cutting edge of science for her classes and thought it would be a fantastic idea to ask Professor Dimitri—a PhD-prepared, renowned content expert in their college—to co-facilitate a class with her. During class, however, Professor Dimitri interrupted several times to correct Professor Brown or add to her point, disrupting Professor Brown's train of thought. In the moment, Professor Brown felt diminished in front of the class after this incident but carried on through the duration of the class. Upon further reflection, Professor Brown decided that, even though the stakes were high and she wanted to maintain a good relationship with Professor Dimitri, it was important to address the situation in more detail and come to an agreement about how she would like to be treated in the future.

Example of Using the DESC Model

- **D**escribe: "Thank you for meeting with me, Professor Dimitri. I'd like to discuss the class we recently co-facilitated."
- **E**xpress: "I know you are the leading expert in this area, and I know you want the best for the students. However, when I am interrupted in the middle of class, I feel diminished, and it could begin to affect my relationship with students."
- **S**uggest: "I would like to discuss our expectations of one another when we co-teach classes in the future."
- **C**onsequences: "Can we co-create an agreement regarding how we will co-facilitate classes in the future?"

Objectives: Becoming familiar with the DESC Model to be able to effectively resolve conflicts. Some students may have difficulty identifying alternative solutions or the consensus goal or seeing the consequences. Follow up with a discussion of what was most challenging and most comfortable.

6. Paired Activity: PAAIL Method

Pair up learners and direct them to review the five steps of the PAAIL Method (Clark & Fey, 2020). Using the following narrative, the pair should play the roles and practice using the model to resolve the conflict. Then they should switch roles and practice them again.

Narrative: The Case of the Nursing Student's Aggression About Clinical Placement

Mario is a senior level nursing student eagerly looking forward to his next clinical placement. He has requested placement in the Cardiac Intensive Care Unit (CICU). Mario expects his request to be accepted by his clinical instructor, Professor Taylor, because he has "the grades." Mario is very excited about the pending placement because he believes being assigned to the CICU will eventually lead to being accepted in a CRNA program. When assignments are made, Mario is placed on the orthopedic floor of a hospital several miles from his home. Mario is devastated and angry. He bursts into Professor Taylor's office angrily demanding to have his clinical placement changed to the CICU.

Example of Using the PAAIL Method

Preview: "Mario, we can talk about your clinical placement when you are more composed and prepared to discuss your concerns in a respectful manner."

Advocacy1: "I realize you prefer to be assigned to the CICU; however, placements there are extremely limited. I am confident you will find nurses on the orthopedic unit to be excellent preceptors as well as patient- and student-centered."

Advocacy2: "I believe the orthopedic unit will provide ample learning opportunities."

Inquiry: "What are your thoughts about my rationale for your clinical placement?"

Listen: To learn and understand.

Objectives: Becoming familiar with the PAAIL Method to be able to use listening skills to effectively resolve conflicts. Follow up with a discussion of what was most challenging and most comfortable.

7. Group Activity: Use Cognitive Rehearsal to Address Real-Life Uncivil Situations

CR is a sophisticated learning activity led by a skilled and experienced facilitator and debriefer. The following activity is designed for educators skilled in all steps of CR.

Step 1: After spending time learning about and applying various evidence-based frameworks using pre-written scenarios, participants assemble into small groups of five to six members. Each member should describe an uncivil encounter that has happened in their academic or work environment and share the encounter with their group.

Step 2: The group is directed to select one uncivil encounter from those shared within the group. The group members then select an evidence-based approach to "script" a response to address the uncivil encounter.

Step 3: Members choose roles to act out the encounter and apply their "script." Group members not selected for the role-play will assume the role of observers.

Step 4: The facilitator oversees the role-play and facilitates a comprehensive coaching and debriefing session. Successful facilitator-led debriefing requires creating safe learning spaces for reflection to help identify aspects of the individual and team performance that went well, aspects that need improvement, and effective ways to address future situations. Some examples of debriefing questions include:

1. **For actors:** What was it like to be part of this experience?
2. **For observers:** What was it like to observe the experience? What did you see? What did you hear? What actions might you take in the future given the same situation?
3. **For all** participants and observers:
    a. How would you describe the experience?
    b. What went well, and what would you do again?

c. What did you learn? How might you apply what you have learned in your clinical practice?

d. What might be done differently next time?

Objectives: Demonstrating communication and conflict competence through learner-derived Cognitive Rehearsal.

Reflection

Take the *Clark Conflict Negotiation Challenge* to improve your conflict negotiation skills and build relationships. To begin, consider a conflict you have experienced or are experiencing with a friend, family member, coworker, classmate, neighbor—or anyone you choose. Use the following steps to work through the conflict. Once you have completed the *Clark Conflict Negotiation Challenge*, consider sharing your observations with a trusted colleague, friend, or family member.

1. Briefly describe the situation and identify the individual(s) involved.
2. Highlight the key issues and perceived reason(s) for the conflict.
3. If you addressed the situation, what strategies did you use? Were they effective?
4. Describe how the conversation started, progressed, and ended.
5. Upon reflection, how satisfied are you with the outcome? What are your next steps?
6. If you avoided addressing the situation, what kept you from addressing it?
7. Upon reflection, how satisfied are you with your decision not to address the situation?

Objective: Open personal reflection of the learner's experiences and application of the POWER skills and conflict resolution models. These can be evaluated as short reflective essays or used as discussion starters.

References

Agency for Healthcare Research and Quality. (2021). *TeamSTEPPS® 2.0*. http://teamstepps.ahrq.gov

Caspersen, D. (2014). *Changing the conversation: The 17 principles of conflict resolution*. Penguin Books.

Clark, C. M. (2019). Combining Cognitive Rehearsal, simulation, and evidence-based scripting to address incivility. *Nurse Educator, 44*(2), 64–68.

Clark, C. M., & Fey, M. K. (2020). Fostering civility in learning conversations: Introducing the PAAIL communication strategy. *Nurse Educator, 45*(3), 139–143.

Clark, C. M., & Gorton, K. (2019). Cognitive Rehearsal, HeartMath, and simulation: Interventions to build resilience and address incivility. *Journal of Nursing Education, 58*(12), 690–697.

Gannon, K. M. (2020). *Radical hope: A teaching manifesto*. West Virginia University Press.

Griffin, M. (2004). Teaching cognitive rehearsal as a shield for lateral violence: An intervention for newly licensed nurses. *Journal of Continuing Education in Nursing, 35*, 257–263.

Griffin, M., & Clark, C. M. (2014). Revisiting Cognitive Rehearsal as an intervention against incivility and lateral violence in nursing: 10 years later. *Journal of Continuing Education in Nursing, 45*(12), 535–542.

Language of Caring. (n.d.). *Making caring visible.* https://languageofcaring.org/

Maxfield, D., & Grenny, J. (2017). Crucial moments in healthcare: Patient safety and quality of care impacted by silence around five common workplace issues. *VitalSmarts,* 1–6.

Palfrey, J. (2018). *Safe spaces, brave spaces: Diversity and free expression in education.* MIT Press.

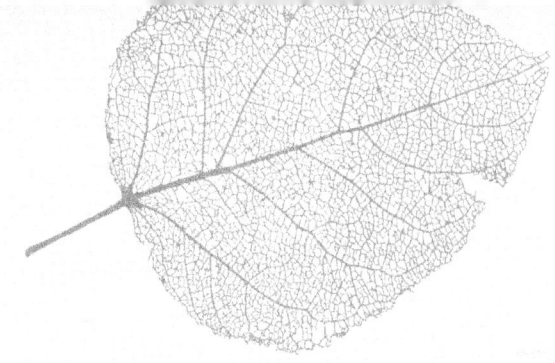

6

The Power of Leadership, Visioning, and Finding Our WHY

LEARNING OUTCOMES

- Describe characteristics of PEAK leaders.
- Identify Kouzes and Posner's Five Practices of Exemplary Leadership.
- Identify Kouzes and Posner's Ten Commitments of Exemplary Leadership.
- Create a personal, professional vision for the future related to nursing and healthcare.
- Craft an individual WHY statement that reflects your life purpose and the difference you wish to make in the world.
- Describe factors associated with an effective mentoring relationship.

Before You Begin

Chapter 6 focuses on the power of leadership and mentoring, crafting a compelling personal professional vision of the future, and discovering and living our purpose, also known as our WHY. Modeling the qualities of PEAK (principled, ethical, authentic, and kind) leadership takes center stage in this chapter. Facilitators are professional role models for learners, and learners are models for one another, as each member explores and applies strategies to strengthen leadership skills and qualities. As Brookfield and Preskill (2016) noted, "nothing produces cynicism quicker [in learners] than the message, 'Do as I say, not as I do'" (p. 6). In other words, walking the talk or practicing what we preach requires facilitators to examine how they demonstrate the behaviors of authentic leadership as well as modeling the positive attributes of the nursing profession.

For facilitators to be respected and viewed as professional role models by learners requires a deepened sense of self and one's aptitude as a leader. Modeling civility and PEAK leadership skills involves an honest appraisal of who we are and how we are viewed by others. Facilitators (and learners) consistently send messages and clues as to what might be considered acceptable behaviors and influence others through leading by example. Thus, being cognizant of our actions and their impact on the learning environment is an essential leadership skill.

Since facilitators of civility and leadership content rely on role-modeling as an instructional tool, the ideal facilitator is someone trusted by learners, possessing a skilled ability to ask probing questions and generate meaningful discussion. These skills are particularly important when assisting learners in developing their personal professional vision of the future and crafting their individual WHY statements. Brookfield (2017) noted that *how* class is facilitated (the way we act and treat learners) is often more important than *what* specific content we impart related to the course—and that facilitator role-modeling is crucial to helping learners think more critically and deeply. In other words, before asking learners to unearth and share their perceptions and experiences, facilitators must demonstrate that they are willing to do the same. Facilitators are encouraged to share their individual WHY statements when leading the learning activities contained in this chapter to role-model a well-thought-out WHY statement for learners.

Crafting a meaningful personal professional vision of a desired future requires thoughtful introspection, time, and asking ourselves some very important and probing questions. The most effective facilitators have identified and ultimately committed to a set of unwavering principles, values, and daily habits. Clarifying principles and values helps us become more self-aware, make ethically-based decisions, set goals, prioritize roles and responsibilities, and serve as leaders, role models, and mentors. There are several excellent tools to clarify principles and values. One example includes the Values Exercise by Kouzes and Pozner (2012). This exercise help to identify principles and values; however, discussing and clarifying your principles and values with a trusted mentor is another great way to solidify your firm beliefs (Clark, 2017). A vision must also be written down, shared, and articulated aloud. As Sinek (2017) noted, "Your vision is only actionable if you say it out loud. If you keep it to yourself, it will remain a figment of your imagination" (p. 5).

Mentoring is akin to positive role-modeling. As facilitators, you will be viewed as leaders and mentors by learners, and this status comes with important responsibilities, including sharing knowledge and experience, guiding the professional development of learners, and inviting multiple viewpoints within a context of mutual respect and trust. Mentoring relationships are characterized by collegiality and collaboration and centered on promoting personal, professional growth. Facilitators can encourage learners to seek out strong and influential mentors to guide their professional career and to also "pay it forward" by mentoring others.

Key Concepts

After reading the chapter, ask the learners to test their understanding of the concepts with short answers.

1. Identify the four characteristics of a PEAK leader.

    Answer: PEAK leaders are principled, ethical, authentic, and kind.

2. Define the four characteristics of a PEAK leader.

    Answer:

    - Being **principled** means using principles and values to build trust and respect, guide decisions, and determine direction to help others, especially in turbulent times.
    - Being **ethical** means taking the right and honorable course of action rather than what is most convenient or in one's own self-interest.
    - Being **authentic** means evaluating goals, core values, and motives and appreciating the impact one has on others.
    - Being **kind** means leading compassionately and seeing kindness as a sign of strength and moral courage.

3. Identify the Five Practices of Exemplary Leadership according to Kouzes and Posner as referenced in Chapter 6.

    Answer: The five practices of exemplary leadership are: 1) modeling the way, 2) inspiring a shared vision, 3) challenging the process, 4) enabling others to act, and 5) encouraging the heart.

4. Identify the Ten Commitments of Exemplary Leadership according to Kouzes and Posner as referenced in Chapter 6.

    Answer:

    1. Clarify values by finding your voice and affirming shared ideas.
    2. Set the example by aligning actions with shared values.

3. Envision the future by imagining exciting and ennobling possibilities.

4. Enlist others in a common vision by appealing to shared aspirations.

5. Search for opportunities by looking outward for innovative ways to improve.

6. Experiment and take risks by constantly generating small wins and learning from experience.

7. Foster collaboration by building trust and facilitating relationships.

8. Strengthen others by increasing self-determination and developing competence.

9. Recognize contributions by showing appreciation for individual excellence.

10. Celebrate values and victories by creating a spirit of community.

5. What are three important developmental activities discussed in Chapter 6 that can help one grow as a leader in nursing and healthcare?

    Answer: Crafting a vision of the future, finding our WHY, and engaging in mentorship and lifelong learning.

6. According to the literature, identify three factors related to effective mentoring.

    Answer:

    1. Mentors and mentees establish a common understanding regarding mentoring practices.

    2. Mentoring success is dependent on the quality of the mentoring relationship.

    3. In addition to financial and administrative support, the organization provides ongoing assistance for a comprehensive mentoring program, training, and matching.

Rationale for Implementation

After reading the chapter, ask the learners to test their understanding of the concepts with short answers.

1. Why is it important to exemplify the characteristics of a PEAK leader in nursing and healthcare?

    Answer: Leaders in nursing and healthcare who exude an approach that integrates being principled, ethical, authentic, and kind can better establish strong relationships built on trust, respect, and a shared desire to take the most ethical and compassionate course of action.

2. Why is it important to craft a personal, professional vision for the future?

   Answer: Crafting a vision for the future helps motivate nurse leaders and others to find meaning in their lives, be their best, and share enthusiasm for their purpose with others. A well-defined vision means knowing your true north; being clear about your values, mission, and purpose; and using your vision to provide guidance and direction during challenging times.

3. Why is it important to find our individual WHY?

   Answer: Leaders in nursing and healthcare who can articulate their WHY can help themselves and others overcome temporary obstacles and difficulties that might otherwise deter them from continuing in their long-term career path. Most people can describe *what* they do and *how* they do it, but only a few individuals can clearly describe *why* they do what they do. WHY statements are powerful declarations that boldly articulate our purpose, unique contribution, and the desired impact of our contribution.

4. Why is it important to engage in mentorship and lifelong learning in nursing and healthcare?

   Answer: Mentorship in nursing and healthcare helps impart wisdom from mentor to mentee, helping both in different capacities, and helps advance the nursing and healthcare professions. The mentor helps guide the mentee from a more experienced background in nursing and healthcare, with consideration to the mentee's specific needs. The process of mentorship creates meaning for both mentors and mentees in their careers and other aspects of their personal and professional lives.

Application of the Concepts

Working in pairs, instruct learners to complete the following exercises.

1. Paired Activity: Crafting a Personal, Professional Vision for the Future

Provide learners with 15 minutes of in-class time to answer the following questions in relation to their personal, professional vision of their career in nursing and healthcare. Then, provide 15 minutes for learners to pair up and share their answers with a colleague in the session. To conclude, ask each pair to share one insightful takeaway they both gained from this learning experience.

1. How would I like others to describe me, my role, and my contributions in nursing and healthcare?

2. What legacy or indelible footprint do I aspire to leave during my career and upon retirement?

3. What aspects of my career bring me the most gratification and meaning?

2. Paired Activity: Creating and Sharing Your Individual WHY Statement

Because this is a topic requiring additional introspection about oneself and career, provide learners with the instructions and questions associated with the activity prior to class. This will give learners time to think critically about their proposed individual WHY statement and discuss it with a trusted friend, mentor, colleague, or family member. During class, provide learners with 15 minutes to share what they learned from that activity with a colleague in the group. Then, ask learners to reconvene as a larger group to share major takeaway points.

1. Using Sinek's template, create your individual WHY statement:

   TO (contribution)_____ SO THAT (impact)_____.

2. Share your individual WHY with a trusted friend, mentor, colleague, or family member.

3. With another colleague during an in-class learning session, discuss the following:
   - What did you learn from the process of creating a WHY statement?
   - What feedback did you receive about your WHY statement?

4. With the larger group, discuss the following question: What is the most important point you learned from creating an individual WHY statement and having it reviewed by a trusted friend, mentor, colleague, or family member?

Reflection

It is important for learners to periodically reflect and build upon their individual WHY statement since a well-developed WHY statement provides guidance and direction during turbulent times. One example of recent turbulence is the challenges faced during the COVID-19 pandemic. Keeping a thoughtful focus on the WHY can help sustain motivation to fulfill a larger purpose in nursing and healthcare. To continue to build their WHY statements, tell learners to mark their calendars to revisit the following questions one to two months after completing this exercise.

1. Revisit your WHY statement. Is there anything about your WHY statement you would like to change? Why or why not? If you revised your WHY statement, write it down.

2. What barriers do you perceive may impact your ability to achieve your WHY? How can these barriers be addressed?

3. What strengths do you have to achieve your WHY? Is there anything further you can do to bolster these strengths?

Facilitator tip: Once learners have created and revisited their individual WHY, have them share their insights with a trusted colleague, friend, or family member.

References

Brookfield, S. D. (2017). *Becoming a critically reflective teacher*. John Wiley & Sons.

Brookfield, S. D., & Preskill, S. (2016). *The discussion book: 50 ways to get people talking*. Jossey-Bass.

Clark, C. M. (2017). *Creating and sustaining civility in nursing education* (2nd ed.). Sigma Theta Tau International.

Kouzes, J. M., & Posner, B. Z. (2012). *The leadership challenge workbook* (3rd ed.). John Wiley & Sons.

Sinek, S. (2017). *Find your why: A practical guide to discovering purpose for you or your team*. Portfolio/Penguin.

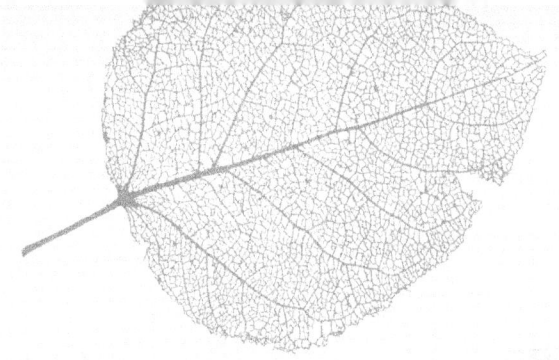

7

Optimizing Self-Care and Professional Well-Being

LEARNING OUTCOMES

- Describe the impact of stress and burnout in nursing and healthcare.
- Discuss the relationship between stress and incivility in nursing and healthcare.
- Identify contributors and outcomes to high stress in nursing practice and nursing education using the Conceptual Model for Fostering Civility in Nursing Education and the Conceptual Model for Fostering Civility in Nursing Education Adapted for Practice.
- Use the Personal Health Assessment to establish a baseline of personal well-being.
- Define change, transition, and the three stages an individual experiences during change according to the Bridges Transition Model.
- Identify at least three strategies to help manage external stress in nursing and healthcare that could affect individual well-being if left unaddressed.
- Discuss the role of resilience through mindfulness in managing stress.
- Implement at least one self-care exercise from Chapter 7 and evaluate its effectiveness.

Before You Begin

Chapter 7 highlights the detrimental impact of stress and burnout, details the relationship between stress and incivility, and provides an abundance of wellness and self-care strategies. While stress is a normal reaction to everyday pressures, at times, stress levels can reach unhealthy levels, disrupt ability to function, and exceed an individual's ability to cope effectively. While nurses and healthcare professionals have always experienced varying levels of workplace stress, the prevalence and novelty of COVID-19, along with its highly infectious variants, have placed unprecedented demands on nurses and healthcare professionals worldwide and caused significant disruption in nearly all aspects of life. Prior to the COVID-19 pandemic, burnout rates for healthcare professionals were already a serious problem. Unfortunately, the pandemic brought additional stressors, which increased the potential for heightened levels of anxiety and burnout.

Facilitators of content related to stress, burnout, exhaustion, and compassion fatigue can begin by looking inward and evaluating their own quality of general health and well-being by completing the Personal Health Assessment contained in Chapter 7. Poorly managed stress and ineffective coping can have detrimental impacts on all domains of wellness and lead to acts of incivility and other workplace aggressions. Carello & Thompson (2021) suggest that facilitators conduct a deep self-reflection to examine their own challenges and vulnerabilities, particularly in light of the COVID-19 pandemic and its effects. The authors further suggest implementing trauma-informed teaching and learning strategies to foster learner engagement.

Integrating healthy coping and self-care strategies into our daily lives is essential to our overall health and well-being. Ashcraft and Gatto (2018, p. 140) describe self-care "as deliberate decisions made, and actions taken by individuals to address their own health and well-being." This assertion suggests that all individuals are empowered to manage their behaviors and resulting health and well-being.

It is also important for facilitators to reinforce the undeniable link between stress and incivility. Increased stress levels, rising tensions, and short tempers can lead to acts of incivility and other workplace aggressions. Whether measured quantitively, qualitatively, or conducting mixed-methodology or biomarker studies, the impact of stress and incivility on worker and patient health and safety is well documented. Skilled facilitators can discuss the connection between stress and incivility and urge learners to implement self-care strategies to mitigate its effects.

Skilled facilitators can identify their own self-care practices and wellness activities. Role-modeling and speaking honestly about your challenges and successes with implementing a self-care program encourages learners to do the same. Consider beginning class with a self-care activity such as a mindfulness practice, deep breathing, or a self-scalp massage. Facilitators may also ask a learner or small group of learners to lead a self-care or wellness exercise at the beginning, during, or at the end of class. There are several examples contained in Chapter 7—or facilitators and learners can implement one of their own. Facilitators and learners are encouraged to create a personal self-care toolkit and implement strategies on a frequent, if not daily, basis.

Due to the sensitive nature of the content (stress, burnout, incivility), implementing various teaching-learning strategies throughout class discussion can help identify challenges learners may be experiencing. For example, pausing for two to three minutes after facilitating 20 to 30 minutes of course content and encouraging learners to discuss and review content in pairs or small groups helps support learning and understanding of the course material and the way it is organized and presented. Pausing also provides learners with an opportunity to review course content and ask clarifying questions (Nilson, 2016). Using clickers or polling apps to pose questions to learners and instantaneously collecting and viewing responses from the entire class is another effective way to facilitate class and generate discussion.

Key Concepts

After reading the chapter, ask the learners to test their understanding of the concepts with short answers.

1. Describe the impact of stress in nursing and healthcare.

    Answer: High stress can lead to confusion, frustration, and fear. Poorly managed stress can lead to poor self-care habits (e.g., diminished motivation to exercise or eat healthy foods). Stress related to the COVID-19 pandemic has caused significant disruption in the economy, at work, and in academic settings, relationships, and healthcare.

2. Define how stress relates to burnout.

    Answer: Increased stress can lead to *burnout*, which can be defined as a condition characterized by long-term exposure to stress and manifested by three classic symptoms: exhaustion, depersonalization (cynicism), and reduced personal accomplishment (Maslach & Leiter, 2016).

3. How does stress relate to incivility in nursing and healthcare?

    Answer: Heightened levels of stress can contribute to increased incivility and other acts of workplace aggression in nursing and healthcare.

4. According to the Conceptual Model for Fostering Civility in Nursing Education Adapted for Practice (Clark, 2017), identify contributors to stress in nursing practice.

    Answer: Answers should include several of the following:

    - Health concerns about self and others
    - Patients with high levels of acuity
    - Increased workloads
    - Staff and equipment shortages
    - Fatigue and moral distress

- Organizational stress and volatility
- Unclear roles and expectations
- Power imbalances
- A lack of knowledge and skills in conflict management

5. According to the Conceptual Model for Fostering Civility in Nursing Education (Clark, 2017), identify contributors to stress in nursing education.

   Answer: Answers should include several of the following:

   - Health concerns about self and others
   - Societal, political, and financial tensions
   - Fear and uncertainty
   - Demanding workloads and juggling multiple roles
   - Technology overload/screen fatigue
   - Organizational stress and volatility
   - Remoteness and isolation
   - A lack of knowledge and skills in managing conflict

6. Describe the meaning of change and transition according to Bridges and the three stages an individual experiences during change according to the Bridges Transition Model (William Bridges Associates, n.d.).

   Answer: *Change* is the external event or situation that takes place. *Transition* is the inner psychological process that individuals go through as they internalize and come to terms with the change. The three stages of change according to the Bridges Transition Model are 1) ending what currently is, 2) a neutral phase in which new roles are learned, and 3) new beginnings that include a renewed sense of purpose to promote successful changes.

7. Identify the four health domains that can be measured using the Gourgouris and Apostolopoulos (2020) Personal Health Assessment.

   Answer: The Personal Health Assessment measures physical, mental, emotional, and spiritual health.

8. Identify and describe at least three strategies to help manage external stress in nursing and healthcare.

   Answer: Stress can be managed through cognitive behavioral therapy (CBT), cognitive reframing, self-affirmations, mirror work, and physical activity.

- CBT is stopping or replacing negative or harmful thoughts with positive thoughts.
- Cognitive reframing is thinking about a situation from another point of view to see a situation from multiple perspectives.
- Positive affirmations include thinking of a positive thought, writing it down, and repeating it several times a day.
- Mirror work can include stating a positive affirmation to oneself in the mirror to experience how this feels and to reflect upon those feelings.
- Physical activity includes exercising, joining online exercise classes, dancing to music, standing up to work, and doing stretching exercises.

9. Define resilience and mindfulness.

   Answer: *Resilience* is the extent to which one can manage, adapt, and recover during or after challenging situations and build capacity to successfully manage future challenges. *Mindfulness* is being fully present, aware of our actions, and not being overwhelmed by external influences.

10. Identify habits to cultivate mindfulness to integrate into an everyday routine.

    Answer: Examples of habits to promote mindfulness include deep breathing, noticing one's surroundings through the five senses, practicing being present and deep breathing while washing one's hands, doing a self-scalp massage, and expressing gratitude.

Rationale for Implementation

After reading the chapter, ask the learners to test their understanding of the concepts with short answers.

1. Why is it important to manage stress in academic and practice settings?

   Answer: Unmanaged stress stemming from practice and academic settings can result in a culture of incivility if remedies, encounters, and opportunities for engagement are missed, avoided, or poorly managed.

2. Why is it important for individuals to assess their personal health?

   Answer: Conducting a personal health assessment can be the basis of establishing a personal self-care and wellness plan. It is essential to establish a starting point for determining next steps in creating a plan to build well-being and personal resilience.

3. During a stressful event, what happens to the brain at the biological level, and why is it important for sound cognition to manage stress?

   Answer: During a stressful event, the amygdala (part of the limbic system and the emotional center of the brain) sends a distress signal to the hypothalamus to activate the stress response.

The amygdala helps control reactions to stress and regulates emotions such as anxiety, aggression, and fear. Calming the amygdala empowers us to think, act, and respond in the most efficient way possible and ultimately heightens our resilience.

Application of the Concepts

Working in small groups, instruct learners to complete the following exercises.

1. Reflection and Sharing Activity: Creating Personal Positive Affirmations for Professional Development

Before leading this activity, reflect on some of your current or past challenges. Have you used positive affirmations to manage your thoughts about these challenges? Why or why not? Journal your thoughts if it would help before leading this session. To help break the ice about this topic, briefly share your reflections about the use of positive affirmations to manage stress with learners at the beginning of the session. Provide 15 minutes for learners to develop one or two positive affirmations that are tailored to their professional development in nursing and healthcare. Then, ask learners to pair up, create, and share their positive affirmations and discuss their feelings after practicing saying their positive affirmations.

1. Create a positive affirmation tailored to helping you grow as a professional in nursing or healthcare. One example could be, "I am letting go of negative thoughts. I will embrace opportunities to continue growing and developing as a professional." Write your positive affirmation down for the next steps.

2. Share your positive affirmation with a trusted colleague, friend, family member, or fellow learner. Discuss what makes this affirmation important to your professional development.

3. Then, take turns saying your positive affirmation out loud or silently in your mind.

4. Discuss how you felt after practicing saying your positive affirmation. Is there anything you would change about your positive affirmation? Why or why not?

2. Group Activity: Creating Expressions of Gratitude

Provide learners with 15 minutes to think about their accomplishments and create a gratitude statement about people, organizations, or resources who helped them achieve their accomplishments. Then, ask learners to share their gratitude statement with a partner. Encourage learners to share their gratitude statement in an email or in person outside of the learning session to the person for whom they are grateful.

1. Think about goals you have accomplished in the past month in your professional role as a nurse or healthcare professional, no matter how large or small. Did anyone help you along the way to accomplish your goals? Did you have access to resources to accomplish your goals that, if not

present, would have otherwise made it much more difficult to achieve goals? Then, take notes about your accomplishments in the past month and people and resources who helped you achieve these accomplishments.

2. Create a gratitude statement about people who helped you achieve your accomplishments, thanking them for their contributions.

3. Take turns sharing your statement of gratitude with a small group of learners.

4. How did you feel after sharing your gratitude statement? Offer feedback to other learners about their gratitude statements.

5. Since sharing your gratitude statement with a group of learners, is there anything you would change about your approach to creating and sharing a gratitude statement? Why or why not?

6. Share your gratitude statement with the person who helped you achieve your goals in an email or in person outside of the learning session.

Reflection

Ask learners to reflect upon the gratitude statements they created and how they felt after sharing their gratitude statements with the person for whom they are grateful.

1. Reflect about the response you received from the person for whom you were grateful. How did the other person respond? How did you feel after sharing your gratitude statement? If you were stressed before sharing this statement, how did you feel in terms of being stressed after you shared your gratitude statement?

2. Since sharing your gratitude statement, is there anything you would like to change or add to your approach? Why or why not?

Facilitator tip: Once learners have reflected about the impact of their gratitude statements, have them share their insights with a trusted colleague, friend, or family member.

References

Ashcraft, P. F., & Gatto, S. L. (2018). Curricular interventions to promote self-care in prelicensure nursing students. *Nurse Educator, 43*(3), 140–144. doi.org/10.1097/NNE.0000000000000450

Carello, J., & Thompson, P. (Eds.). (2021). *Lessons from the pandemic: Trauma-informed approaches to college, crisis, and change.* Palgrave Macmillan.

Clark, C. M. (2017). *Creating and sustaining civility in nursing education* (2nd ed.). Sigma Theta Tau International Honor Society of Nursing.

Gourgouris, E., & Apostolopoulos, K. (2020). *7 keys to navigating a crisis: A practical guide to emotionally dealing with pandemics & other disasters.* The Happiness Center.

Maslach, C., & Leiter, M. P. (2016). Understanding the burnout experience: Recent research and its implications for psychiatry. *World Psychiatry, 15*(2), 103–111. https://doi.org/10.1002/wps.20311

Nilson, L. B. (2016). *Teaching at its best: A research-based resource for college instructors* (4th ed.). Jossey-Bass.

William Bridges Associates. (n.d.). *Bridges Transition Model.* https://wmbridges.com/about/what-is-transition/

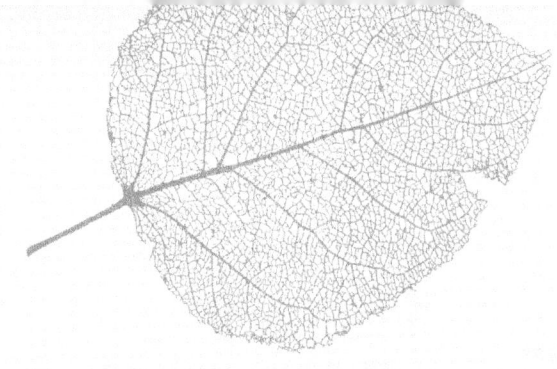

8

Leadership Support and Raising Awareness for Organizational Change

LEARNING OUTCOMES

- Define the Pathway for Fostering Organizational Civility (PFOC).
- Explain how organizational behavior informs the process of fostering organizational change for civility according to the PFOC.
- Illustrate the difference between buy-in and ownership in supporting change initiatives to foster organizational civility.
- Describe the role of organizational leadership in fostering civility and health work environments.
- Discuss how to enlist leadership support and raise awareness (Step 1 of the PFOC).
- Discuss strategies to assess the organizational culture (Step 2 of the PFOC).

Before You Begin

Chapter 8 focuses on implementing steps 1 and 2 of the Pathway for Fostering Organizational Civility (PFOC), tools to measure workplace health, and the essential role of leadership in fostering civility and healthy work environments. Facilitators of this content are urged to become familiar with the role of leadership and followership within dynamic systems, cultural transformation, systems theory, and theoretical frameworks to effect and sustain organizational change.

The PFOC provides a comprehensive, evidence-based, eight-step systematic approach to foster and sustain organizational change. Chapter 8 focuses on the first two steps: 1) enlisting leadership support and raising awareness, and 2) assessing the organizational culture. Transforming the workplace culture can be a heavy lift for many organizations since it is often time-, resource-, and labor-intensive. Even when managed well, change is frequently viewed as undesirable and unwanted. Further, people involved in the change, especially those perceived to be most impacted by the change, may be reluctant to speak up and voice their concerns.

Before facilitating class, think about a time when you experienced a major change in your work environment. If you are an academic nurse educator, perhaps you led the team charged with developing and implementing a comprehensive curriculum change. If you are a nurse manager, perhaps you were part of a team responsible for writing and implementing a no-visitor policy during the peak of the COVID-19 pandemic. Reflect upon your own thoughts, feelings, and outlook about the change. Did you feel threatened by the impending change? Did you have feelings of resistance or resentment? Or perhaps you felt energized and excited about the change. Despite how you felt about the change, how did you participate in it? Did you take an active role? Did you lead the change? Did you raise important questions about the change? Reflecting on your thoughts about and responses to a major change—and characterizing the outcomes (both constructive and undesirable)—can be a great way to start class and facilitate the Chapter 8 learning activities.

Because Chapter 8 reinforces the essential role of leadership in fostering healthy work environments, facilitators are advised to consider their personal and professional experiences with leaders as well as their own leadership style. Contemplate how different leadership styles influence positive employee engagement and productive involvement in major change initiatives. Did leaders strive for employee buy-in or ownership for the change? Did one or the other make a perceptible difference in how employees participated or resisted the change?

Next, think about theories of organizational change. When undergoing a major change in your workplace, did your organizational leaders use a change theory or framework for planned change? If so, which theory was used? Did members of the organization find the theory helpful as a road map for change? If a change theory was used to effect transformational change, how does the theory compare with the PFOC? Were there champions engaged to motivate the change?

Lastly, ponder the swift and immediate changes that occurred in healthcare stemming from the COVID-19 pandemic and its myriad manifestations. Which changes impacted you and your colleagues most? Which changes are still in place, which changes have been abandoned, and which changes still need to be implemented? What was your role in effecting or suggesting these changes? How do you assess your energy level to participate in these changes? How motivated are you to lead others as changes are made?

Intentionally reflecting on the many and varied questions noted in this section is important for facilitators. Being thoughtful and contemplative about your personal experiences with change helps strengthen the skills needed for effective facilitation regarding the PFOC, the importance of a theoretical approach to change, and understanding the role of leadership in fostering healthy work environments. Prestia (2020) reminds us that nurse leaders must combine the critical elements of self-awareness and reflection to effectively monitor our moral compasses. Similarly, Rosenbaum et al. (2018) noted that storytelling, sensemaking, and reflection play a positive role in leadership development and change management.

Key Concepts

After reading the chapter, ask the learners to test their understanding of the concepts with short answers.

1. Define the Pathway for Fostering Organizational Civility (PFOC) and the first two steps of the PFOC.

   Answer: The PFOC is an eight-step evidence-based approach to foster and sustain organizational change. The first two steps of the model are: 1) enlisting leadership support and raising awareness, and 2) assessing the organizational culture.

2. Describe unique aspects of organizational behavior that influence change and transformation.

   Answer: Organizations are continually evolving, adapting through the multiple channels of communications and interactions between and among individuals and teams that become the impetus for change and transformation.

3. Explain the difference between *buy-in* and *ownership* in asking for support from organizational leaders about implementing a civility and health work environment initiative.

   Answer: One example of *buy-in* would be convincing others to accept an idea that has been developed. In contrast, facilitating *ownership* involves members of all levels of the organization at the beginning of a change initiative and allows them to take an active role in the design and implementation of an initiative. It is more effective to facilitate ownership for a civility and healthy work environment initiative so that key stakeholders have collective responsibility for developing and executing the change.

4. Describe the importance of organizational leadership in fostering workplace civility.

   Answer: Leadership support at all levels, especially executive level support, is essential for transformational and sustained organizational change. Executive level leaders possess a broader view of workplace issues, wider span of influence, and can provide resources (human, financial, time, technology) so the work can be done. Having leadership on board is pivotal to successful workplace transformation. Establishing a civility champion who is a well-respected leader who also has a role in administration in the organization is an excellent strategy to inspire and encourage other leaders and managers to commit to an organizational civility initiative.

5. Discuss one method to enlist leadership support and raise awareness as Step 1 of the PFOC.

   Answer: Raising awareness about the detrimental effects of incivility and other workplace aggressions with organizational leaders can be achieved through sharing data points about its harmful effects through various modes of communication.

6. Discuss strategies to assess the organizational culture as Step 2 of the PFOC.

   Answer: Assessing the organizational culture can be achieved by administering one of six assessment tools described in Chapter 8 to people within an organization. These six tools include:

   1. American Association of Critical-Care Nurses Healthy Work Environment Tool
   2. Workplace Incivility/Civility Survey
   3. Workplace Relational Civility Scale
   4. Civility, Respect, Engagement in the Workforce Scale
   5. Negative Acts Questionnaire – Revised
   6. Healthy Work Environment Inventory

   Analyzing information from formal and informal reports, satisfaction surveys, regulatory reports, interviews, focus groups, and open forums can augment the formal assessment information. Maintaining and assuring confidentiality and integrity of the assessment data and upholding all human subject protocols are critical.

Rationale for Implementation

After reading the chapter, ask the learners to test their understanding of the concepts with short answers.

1. Why is it important to gain the support of organizational leaders to implement civility and health work environment initiatives?

   Answer: Transformational and sustained change requires broad-based collaboration. Teams and individuals need support from leaders to provide needed resources to foster civility and healthy work environment initiatives.

2. Why is it important to assess the work environment using one of the organizational culture measurement tools provided in Chapter 8?

   Answer: Each organization has a unique history and culture. Thorough assessment of the organizational culture is needed to identify areas of strength and excellence as well as areas for growth and improvement. Assessment of the organizational culture can yield meaningful information to develop and implement a system-wide, data-driven action plan to individualize the civility initiative, thus increasing the chance of success.

Application of the Concepts

Working with partners, instruct learners to complete the following exercises.

1. Role-Play Activity: Using Role-Play to Practice Enlisting Leadership Support and Raising Awareness for Fostering Civility in the Workplace

For this activity, ask learners to use role-play and partner with another person. Provide learners with up to 30 minutes for each person to complete their script in 15 minutes, and then the remainder of the time to act out and discuss the scenario. The role-play can be repeated with partners switching roles. Encourage learners to take turns and then debrief about their experiences.

1. Using the information presented on pages 134 to 138 about civility in the workplace, harmful effects of incivility, benefits of civility, and civility in healthcare, create a brief script or bullet-pointed outline to act out (role-play) being an employee who secured a meeting with a high-level executive individual or team to advocate for organizational attention and resources to develop and implement a healthy work environment initiative.

Example Template

- Brief introduction of the problem (i.e., workplace incivility), benefits of civility and healthy work environments
- Data points to illustrate the problem
- Proposed action and resources needed to foster healthy work environments

2. Use the script to provide the person acting in the role of an executive with an overview of the problem, data to illustrate the problem, data to support benefits of civility, and proposed actions needed to foster healthy work environment. One learner will play the role of an executive listening, and the other will use their composed script.

3. Once the script is delivered, ask your partner for feedback. Is there anything you would edit or add to the script? Why or why not?

2. Paired Activity: Comparing and Contrasting Tools to Assess the Organizational Culture

Encourage learners to pair up and compare the six different tools discussed in Chapter 8 to measure the health of an organization's culture and work environment. Learners may also wish to conduct an internet search for other relevant tools or suggest a tool that learners have used in their workplace. Provide learner pairs with up to 20 minutes to exchange their thoughts about the assessment tools. Describe how this activity relates to the prior activity, and stress the importance of continuous assessment of an organization's culture to foster civil and healthy work environments.

1. There are six different assessment tools introduced in Chapter 8 to assess the health of an organization's culture and work environment. Ask learners to pair up with a colleague and review the following six assessment tools described on pages 139 to 142 of Chapter 8 and/or conduct an internet search to explore other relevant assessment tools including assessment tools being used in the workplace:

    - American Association of Critical-Care Nurses (AACN) Healthy Work Environment Tool
    - Workplace Incivility/Civility Survey
    - Workplace Relational Civility Scale
    - Civility, Respect, Engagement in the Workforce Scale
    - Negative Acts Questionnaire – Revised
    - Healthy Work Environment Inventory

2. Considering these tools, which one would you select to measure the health and work environment of your organization? Discuss the reasoning for your selection.

3. Were there multiple tools that could be useful for assessing the health of the work environment at your organization? If so, please describe the other tools that could be used and the reasoning for these thoughts.

Reflection

Enlisting leadership support is a first step to assessing the organizational culture to foster a healthier work environment. Reflect on the script you practiced in the role-play to introduce facts and reasons to assess and foster healthier work environments. Next, consider how the tool you selected in the second activity might be integrated into your script and presentation to the executive leadership individual or team.

1. How did you feel while acting in the role of an employee speaking to a high-level executive team or individual about the extent to which workplace incivility is a problem and the importance of healthy work environments? Is there anything you would have changed about your script? Why or why not?

2. Likewise, how did you feel while acting in the role of a high-level executive listening to an employee about the extent to which workplace incivility is a problem and the importance of fostering healthy work environments? What are your thoughts about having a neutral party administer an evidence-based assessment tool to measure the organizational culture? Is there anything you would suggest the other learner to change in their script? Why or why not?

Facilitator tip: Once learners have reflected about scripts to enlist leadership support for fostering organizational attention toward civility and healthy work environments, have them share their insights with a trusted colleague, friend, or family member.

References

Prestia, A. (2020). The moral obligation of nurse leaders. *Nurse Leader, 18*(4), 326–328.

Rosenbaum, D., Taska, L., & More, E. (2018). The role of reflection in planned organizational change. *Change Management: An International Journal, 18*(3–4), 1–22. doi.org/10.18848/2327-798X/CGP/v18i02/1-22

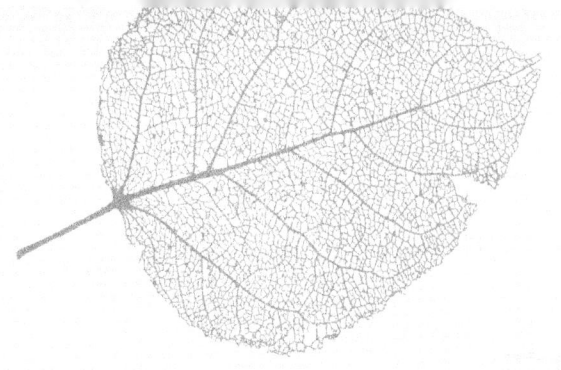

9
Galvanizing a High-Performing Civility Team

LEARNING OUTCOMES

- Specify characteristics of high-performing teams in nursing and healthcare.
- Describe psychological safety as a part of nursing and healthcare team norms.
- Define a Civility Team and state its primary two-fold purpose.
- Identify and describe cultural factors within organizational cultures.
- Discuss how a Civility Team or designee can utilize information gleaned from the organizational assessment to foster a healthy work environment.
- Describe a *golden moment* in your time working on nursing and/or healthcare teams and how it informs your perspectives about your current work situation.

Before You Begin

Chapter 9 focuses on implementing Step 3 of the Pathway for Fostering Organizational Civility (PFOC). This step includes galvanizing and empowering high-performing teams and establishing psychological safety to achieve civility excellence and healthy work environments. To effectively educate learners about the content contained in Chapter 9, facilitators need to be conversant with the characteristics of high-performing teams and specific strategies to build psychological safety between and among team members.

While preparing for class, facilitators can reflect upon the types of teams they have been part of over the years. It can be a work team, sports team, volunteer group, or any other team or committee where the members are dependent on one another to produce results. As you consider your membership on various teams throughout your life, think about the *worst* team experience you have encountered. Which team comes to mind? Take a few minutes to write down the specific traits or characteristics that made the experience negative or undesirable. How did this experience affect you and other members of the team? What lessons did you learn from this experience? How have these lessons impacted your membership on subsequent teams?

Next, think of the *best* team experience you have encountered and write down the specific traits or characteristics that made the experience positive or exceptional. How did this experience affect you and other members of the team? What lessons did you learn from this experience? How have these lessons impacted your membership on subsequent teams? How do the traits or characteristics you identified regarding your *best* team compare with the list of high-performing team competencies displayed in Chapter 9 and in the following sidebar?

Competencies of High-Performing Teams

- Share a common vision, purpose, direction
- Establish and commit to a team charter with team norms
- Foster interpersonal trust and psychological safety
- Utilize effective problem-solving and decision-making skills
- Invite feedback and varying opinions and perspectives
- Focus on process, execution, and achieving results
- Clarify roles for all team members
- Establish and evaluate priorities and interventions
- Utilize constructive communication and conflict negotiation
- Implement objective metrics to measure individual and team performance

Recognizing the traits and characteristics that exemplify high-performing teams helps facilitators coach learners on what makes up a good or excellent team experience and what makes up an inferior or unfavorable team experience. Asking learners to share their personal experiences can enrich the conversation and add meaning to the large group discussion. Facilitators might also consider asking a provocative question or posing a problem to be solved. Because Chapter 9 is focused on high-performing teams and building psychological safety between and among team members, facilitators might pose a probing question to open the dialogue related to both topics and then continue by asking succeeding questions based on learner responses. This type of questioning is referred to as the *Socratic method* or *Socratic questioning*. The following question is an example of a probing question based on the content contained in Chapter 9:

> Drawing from your readings and work experiences, how might nurses and other healthcare professionals promote and ensure psychological safety within care teams?

After posing the question and having learners respond, consider using the Socratic method to mobilize and expand group participation and bring life to course content. The Socratic method is one in which facilitators pose thoughtful questions to help learners think, reflect, and learn—to hone problem-solving and critical thinking skills and improve long-term retention of knowledge (Clark, 2017). The Socratic method is designed to deeply explore the meaning, justification, or strength of a claim or a line of reasoning (Makhene, 2019).

Using the probing question previously mentioned, here are some examples for Socratic questioning:

- Is psychological safety the most important issue to consider when building high-performing teams?
- What are some of the challenges for the healthcare team regarding the complexity of this situation?
- What factors prompted you to support that position?
- Could you elaborate further?
- Can you give us an example?
- How might you verify or test that assumption?
- Could you be more specific?
- How might we look at this in other ways?

Edmondson (1999) first coined the term *psychological safety* and defined it as "a shared belief held by members of a team that the team is safe for interpersonal risk taking and a team climate characterized by interpersonal trust and mutual respect in which people are comfortable being themselves" (p. 354). Edmondson (2019) further noted that psychological safety is present when colleagues trust and respect each other and feel able, even obligated, to be candid. Clark (2020) described psychological safety as a condition in which one feels included, safe to learn, safe to contribute, and safe to challenge the status quo—all without fear of being embarrassed, marginalized, or punished in some way. Achieving and sustaining psychological safety is imperative for high team performance.

Edmondson (2019) provided key questions for team members to consider when assessing a team's level of psychological safety. To gain a better understanding of psychological safety in work teams, facilitators can consider and respond to the following questions (Edmondson, 2019, p. 20) based on their experiences as a member of a current work team. This activity will also be conducted with learners in the Application of the Concepts section of this Facilitator Guide.

1. If you make a mistake on this team, it is often held against you.
2. Members of this team are able to bring up problems and tough issues.
3. People on this team sometimes reject others for being different.
4. It is safe to take a risk on this team.
5. It is difficult to ask other members of this team for help.
6. No one on this team would deliberately act in a way that undermines my efforts.
7. Working with members of this team, my unique skills and talents are valued and utilized.

Intentionally co-creating and collaborating as team members to build and sustain psychologically safe, high-performing teams are critical leadership skills. For respectfully speaking up and advocating for self and others to become routine and psychologically safe, these acts must be supported system-wide and modeled by all members of an organization. Facilitators are in a key position to illuminate and model these important leadership skills that are not only necessary for fostering civility and healthy work environments but also essential for patient and worker safety.

Key Concepts

After reading the chapter, ask the learners to test their understanding of the concepts with short answers.

1. Define and describe a *team*.

    Answer: The World Health Organization (2014) defines a team as a set of two or more people who interact dynamically, interdependently, and adaptively toward a common and valued goal, objective, and/or mission where members have specific roles or functions to perform and have a limited life span of membership. Thus, a team is comprised of a small number of people with complementary skills who are committed and accountable to a common purpose, performance goals, and approach.

2. Describe characteristics of high-performing teams.

    Answer: A high-performing team is a cohesive group of goal-focused individuals with specialized expertise and complementary skills who collaborate, innovate, and produce exceptional results. High-performing teams are highly productive and motivated to achieve a common goal. Members of high-performing teams are clear about their roles and recognize how their efforts align with the organizational mission and vision.

3. Describe psychological safety.

    Answer: *Psychological safety* is defined as a climate in which people are comfortable expressing themselves, a belief that the work environment is safe for interpersonal risk-taking, and a feeling of safety to express relevant ideas, questions, or concerns. Colleagues who are in a psychologically safe climate can ask for help without ridicule.

4. Identify, define, and describe cultural factors to examine as part of a Civility Team's organizational assessment.

    Answer: An organizational cultural analysis involves the examination of factors that influence individual and collective perceptions and reactions to the environment and to proposed changes. Cultural factors include values, norms, organizational support systems, peer support, and climate.

    These factors in an organizational cultural analysis are defined and described as follows:

    - **Values:** Strong beliefs about the appropriate way to behave, including principles and standards that motivate our attitudes and actions. These deeply held principles help shape the foundation for what we believe to be important.
    - **Norms:** Expected and accepted behavior in the workplace. Group expectations of behavior are co-created and accepted.
    - **Organizational support systems:** Laws, rules, policies, procedures, guidelines, and informal communication networks. Formal and informal systems govern the workplace.
    - **Peer support:** Encouragement and collaboration from coworkers who provide support emotionally, mentally, and psychologically. Peer support includes relationship-building, mentoring, role-modeling, a sense of teamwork, and celebrating successes.
    - **Climate:** Working conditions, supervision, and interpersonal relationships. Climate is studied in terms of the extent of a sense of community, a shared vision, and a positive outlook.

5. List the two primary overall functions of Civility Teams.

   Answer: The primary purpose of the Civility Team is two-fold: 1) to support and advance the mission of the healthy work environment initiative, and 2) to oversee the development, implementation, and evaluation of a data-driven action plan.

6. Identify other important functions of the Civility Team.

   Answer:

   - Analyze, organize, and report organizational assessment information
   - Participate in leadership development
   - Appraise individual and team commitment and availability of resources
   - Co-create a team charter with team norms and build in accountability measures
   - Identify empirical measures, assessment strategies, and benchmarks for organizational civility and success
   - Determine resources, timeline, and cost structure for the healthy work environment initiative
   - Garner broad-based support for the healthy work environment initiative

Rationale for Implementation

After reading the chapter, ask the learners to test their understanding of the concepts with short answers.

1. Why is it important to assemble a Civility Team of diverse membership and backgrounds?

   Answer: Members should represent diverse ideas to strengthen the team's understanding of organizational issues at all levels. For example, having members on the team who hold formal leadership roles working with members who do not have formal leadership roles can create a broader shared understanding of organizational processes and practices needing addressing to promote civility.

2. Why is psychological safety a key element of fostering high-performing teams in nursing and healthcare?

   Answer: Psychological safety is critical in high-performing teams in nursing and healthcare because being able to ask questions and report mistakes fosters excellence in outcomes for patients, students, and colleagues. Processes to care for patients can be improved when communication is open, in a psychologically safe environment, between members of the healthcare team.

Application of the Concepts

Working in small groups, instruct learners to complete the following exercises.

1. Group Activity: Creating a Concept Map for High-Performing Teams

Concept mapping is a teaching method used to facilitate critical thinking whereby learners integrate new sub-concepts and related ideas into an existing cognitive structure to foster meaningful learning and provide a visual representation of a concept and sub-concepts and related ideas (Oermann et al., 2018). Provide groups with up to 30 minutes to complete their concept maps. Build in time for each group to share their maps with the larger group.

1. For this activity, assemble into groups of four to five members and place the major concept of high-performing teams in the center of the map. Then build and connect sub-concepts and related ideas to show interrelationships with the major concept of high-performing teams. Following is an example template of a concept map with sub-concepts and related ideas.

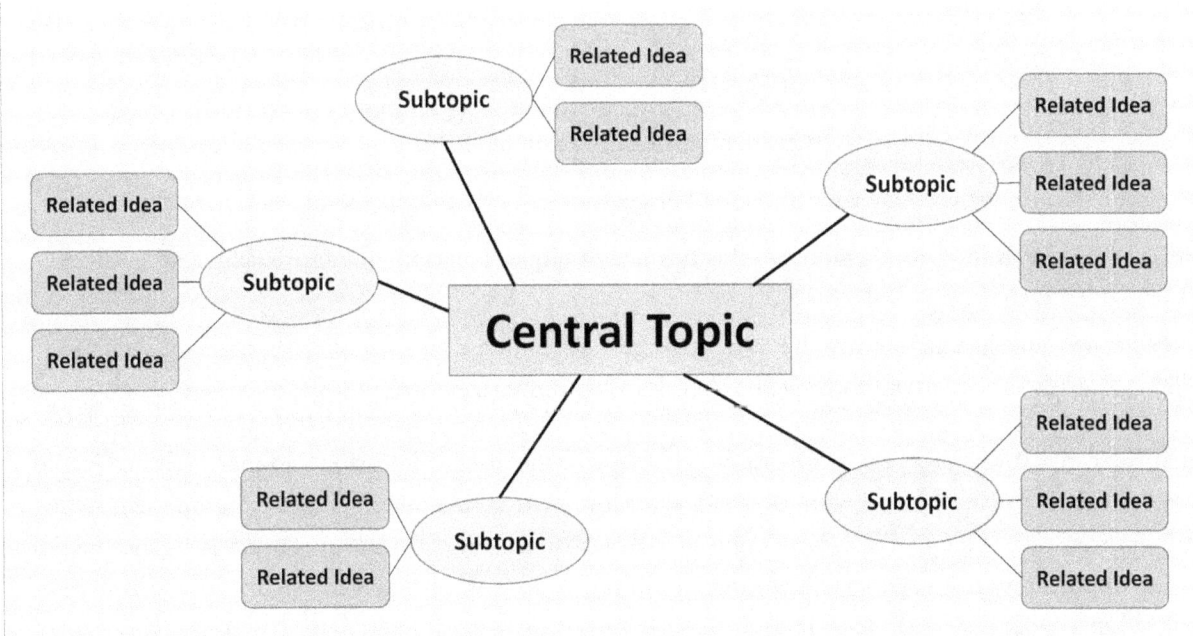

2. Once the concept map is completed, have each group share their map with one or two other groups to discuss similarities and differences.

2. Group Activity: Assessing Psychological Safety in Work Teams

The facilitator will provide an index card numbered 1 to 6 to distribute to learners and ask learners to assemble into groups according to their number. For example, all learners drawing the index card with #1 will assemble into a group, all learners with #2 will assemble into another group, and so on. The goal is to randomly assign learners to groups to increase the potential that group members will be more diverse and from different workplaces and backgrounds.

1. Once learners assemble into groups, learners will be asked to reread pages 152–153 of the text.
2. Then, learners will be asked to reflect upon a group, team, or committee in which they are currently or most recently a member.
3. Learners will be asked to discuss in small groups the seven questions posed by Edmondson (2019, p. 20) listed here as they relate to the group, team, or committee identified in question #2.
   1. If you make a mistake on this team, it is often held against you.
   2. Members of this team are able to bring up problems and tough issues.
   3. People on this team sometimes reject others for being different.
   4. It is safe to take a risk on this team.
   5. It is difficult to ask other members of this team for help.
   6. No one on this team would deliberately act in a way that undermines my efforts.
   7. Working with members of this team, my unique skills and talents are valued and utilized.

Once groups have had an opportunity to discuss these seven questions, a spokesperson from each group will be asked to share a "gem" or a "pearl of wisdom" with the larger group.

Facilitator tip: A *gem* or a *pearl of wisdom* is a synthesis of the group discussion and may be posed in the form of a provocative question, a key concept or discovery, or an interesting idea to engage the class in further discussion. This synthesis is an important aspect of learning. A *synthesis* is not a summary; instead, it is an opportunity to create new knowledge out of existing knowledge and to use this new information to develop a cogent argument or a unique perspective on a broader topic (Clark, 2017).

Reflection

The author defines a *golden moment* as a zestful, dynamic time in our working life when we felt inspired, validated, and filled with a sense of well-being, joy, and delight. Living a golden moment means we are experiencing the incredible joy and satisfaction of being part of a high-performing team engaged in very challenging yet rewarding and meaningful work. Reflect on your career and respond to the following questions:

1. Have you ever experienced a golden moment in your career? Think back to a time (or perhaps it is now in your current workplace) when being a member of a team or committee left you feeling joyful, zestful, and positively unstoppable.

2. What was the experience like? How would you describe it?

3. Rate your golden moment on a scale ranging from 0 to 10 (0 = absolute worst work experience ever to 10 = most incredible work experience ever). If it is truly a golden moment your rating will be 9 or 10/10!

4. As you reflect on your current work situation, if your rating is less than 7 or 8, or even lower, examine whether your current work setting is the right fit for you.

Facilitator tip: Once learners have reflected on their golden moment, have them share their insights with a trusted colleague, friend, or family member.

References

Clark, C. M. (2017). *Creating and sustaining civility in nursing education* (2nd ed.). Sigma Theta Tau International.

Clark, T. R. (2020). *The 4 stages of psychological safety: Defining the path to inclusion and innovation.* Berrett-Koehler.

Edmondson, A. (1999). Psychological safety and learning behavior in work teams. *Administrative Science Quarterly, 44*(2), 350–383. doi.org/10.2307/2666999

Edmondson, A. C. (2019). *The fearless organization: Creating psychological safety in the workplace for learning, innovation, and growth.* John Wiley & Sons.

Makhene, A. (2019). The use of the Socratic inquiry to facilitate critical thinking in nursing education. *Health SA Gesondheid, Journal of Interdisciplinary Health Sciences, 24*(1224), 1–6. doi.org/10.4102/hsag.v24i0.1224

Oermann, M. H., DeGagne, J. C., & Phillips, B. C. (2018). *Teaching in nursing and the role of the educator: The complete guide to best practices in teaching, evaluation, and curriculum development* (2nd ed.). Springer Publishing.

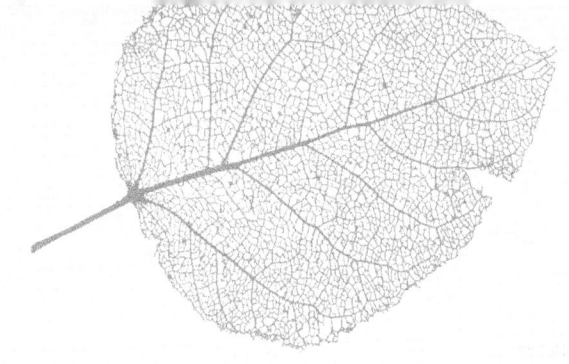

10

Develop, Implement, and Evaluate a Data-Driven Action Plan

LEARNING OUTCOMES

- Identify John Kotter's (1996) elements for creating an organizational vision statement as part of designing a data-driven action plan (Step 4 of the PFOC) to promote organizational civility.

- Discuss the importance of crafting a compelling civility vision statement.

- Define the meaning and purpose of co-creating a Civility Charter and team norms.

- Understand the role of accountability in fulfilling team norms.

- Identify the steps to implement the data-driven action plan (Step 5 of the PFOC).

- Discuss the process for evaluating the data-driven action plan (Step 6 of the PFOC).

Before You Begin

Chapter 10 details Steps 4, 5, and 6 of the Pathway for Fostering Organizational Civility (PFOC). Step 4 involves formulating information gleaned from the organizational culture assessment into a data-driven action plan which is implemented during Step 5 and evaluated during Step 6 of the PFOC. Effective and productive action plans are well developed, efficiently executed, and evaluated on an ongoing basis to measure the effectiveness of interventions and achievement of outcomes. When developing an action plan for civility and healthy work environments, four key elements are highlighted in Chapter 10: generating a compelling vision for the civility initiative, co-creating a Civility Charter with team agreements or norms, implementing a shared or professional governance model, and designing a comprehensive civility education plan. To effectively facilitate learning activities related to these four areas, facilitators are urged to consider their personal and professional experiences with each element.

To prepare for facilitating the learning activities contained in this chapter, begin by accessing and reviewing the foundational documents that undergird and support your current organization. Read and reflect upon the language included in the vision, mission, philosophy, and values statements. Do they accurately reflect a compelling short- and long-term vision of the future? Are the statements energizing and optimizing? Do they inspire action and have an emotional appeal? Do they underscore a commitment to civility, inclusion, and a culture of belonging? Further, are you able to articulate your personal, professional vision of the future and how it relates to the organization where you are employed? In other words, how does your personal, professional vision align or misalign with the vision of your organization? How successful are you in living your personal and organizational vision, mission, and values? And lastly, how are you holding yourself and others accountable to fulfill the organizational statements? These are important aspects to consider when engaging learners in meaningful discussion about the important role that foundational statements play in guiding all members of the organization toward a shared vision of civility, inclusion, and belonging.

Next, consider the utility of having a Civility Charter or Commitment to Coworkers within your own department or work team. Have you and your teammates co-created a charter with team agreements or norms? If so, consider sharing your experience with learners and, in turn, asking them to share their own experiences. How well are the team agreements or norms working to support a civil, healthy work environment? How often are the team agreements or norms discussed, reviewed, and revised when necessary? How are members of the team holding themselves and each other accountable for abiding by the team agreements or norms? For those who have not co-created and collaborated to implement a team charter and norms, be ready to discuss the process with learners and how these documents reinforce an individual and collective commitment to fostering civility and healthy work environments—and provide a touchstone for desired workplace behaviors.

The next topic to consider is the development and implementation of a shared governance or professional governance model in nursing and healthcare. In some organizations, shared governance models have waned during and in the aftermath of the COVID-19 pandemic. Hess et al. (2020) offer advice and lessons learned related to the COVID-19 pandemic and shared governance in American hospitals. Facilitators are well-positioned to generate discussion with learners on this important and relevant topic. Thinking about how the pandemic has influenced shared governance (and vice versa) in your own institution can provide a starting point for discussion with learners.

The fourth and final element for action planning includes designing and implementing a comprehensive civility education plan. Engaging learners in this aspect of the healthy work environment initiative requires facilitators to reinforce the basic features of a comprehensive education plan. For example, a well-developed educational plan provides a detailed road map for reaching critical milestones and maximizes the potential for successfully meeting the goals identified in the healthy work environment initiative. Key areas of inquiry need to be addressed for the civility education plan to be successful, including:

1. How is the educational plan connected and aligned with a) the organizational vision and b) the vision to create and sustain a healthy, civil work environment?
2. What are the guiding principles supporting the educational plan?
3. Is the educational plan supported by empirical evidence and/or best practices?
4. What are the short- and long-term goals of the educational plan? How will they be accomplished? Within which time frame?
5. Who will be responsible for implementing the educational plan?
6. How will the educational plan be successfully rolled out and evaluated?
7. What resources are needed to meet the objectives/outcomes of the educational plan (human, technological, financial, time)?
8. Is there a clear description of the instructional methods and activities needed to ensure the success of the educational plan?
9. What processes need to be implemented to measure the ongoing effectiveness of the educational plan? How will necessary adjustments be made to the educational plan throughout the process?

In April 2022, the National Academy of Medicine (NAM, 2022) announced a national plan for health workforce well-being and resilience. The national plan is focused on several priority areas including establishing positive work and learning environments and organizational cultures. The national plan builds on the National Academies of Sciences, Engineering, and Medicine Report (2019) calling for a systems approach to healthcare professional well-being. Facilitators might consider how these important works provide convincing rationale for developing, implementing, and evaluating data-driven action plans to foster civility and healthy work and learning environments.

Key Concepts

After reading the chapter, ask the learners to test their understanding of the concepts with short answers.

1. List the six elements needed for an organizational vision statement according to Kotter (1996).

    Answer: There are six elements of a vision statement, according to Kotter, including 1) inspiring image of the future, 2) creating long-term interests that appeal to employees and stakeholders, 3) designing realistic and attainable goals, 4) providing adequate clarity to guide decision-making, 5) planning a flexible response to changing conditions, and 6) communicating a message easily.

2. List the eight steps to Latham's (1995) framework to create an organizational vision statement.

    Answer: The eight steps to Latham's framework are: 1) collect input, 2) brainstorm, 3) shrink the mess, 4) develop the rough draft, 5) refine the statement, 6) test the criteria, 7) obtain approval, and 8) communicate and celebrate.

3. Define a *Civility Charter* and its purpose.

    Answer: A Civility Charter is defined by the author as a pledge or a commitment to coworkers whereby all members of the organization commit to fostering civility and a healthy work environment that promotes respect, teamwork, professionalism, and inclusion.

4. Define the meaning of *team norms*.

    Answer: Team norms, also called ground rules, team agreements, social contracts, or rules of engagement, are a set of guidelines that a group co-creates to structure the interactions of group members with one another.

5. Define accountability.

    Answer: As defined by Bregman (2016), accountability is upheld when a commitment is delivered, responsibility for an outcome is assumed, and initiative to follow through on a commitment is taken.

6. Define and explain the purpose of *shared governance* in practice and in education.

    Answer: In nursing practice, shared governance provides nurses with input over their practice, input into what is needed to provide quality patient care, and opportunities to make decisions related to staffing, policy and procedure development, resource acquisition and utilization, innovation, and research (Hess et al., 2020).

    Shared governance (aka professional governance) in nursing education is defined as "an accountability-based, dynamic partnership among leadership, faculty, and staff, founded on equity, empowerment, and shared decision-making to improve the quality of services provided and work life within the academic learning environment (Boswell et al., 2017, p. 201).

7. As part of a Civility Education Plan, what are the three types of workshops the Civility Team could facilitate to foster a shared understanding and motivation for achieving greater organizational civility?

    Answer: The three types of workshops in a civility education plan include a focus on 1) understanding the importance of civility, 2) identifying the focus of improving civility after conducting an organizational cultural assessment, and 3) transforming the organization through agreeing to meaningful and achievable goals to improve civility at the individual, team, and organizational levels.

8. What steps are included in a data-driven action plan? (Step 5 of the PFOC)

    Answer: 1) Identify specific, measurable interventions; 2) prioritize interventions based on urgency and importance; 3) establish clear timelines and responsibilities; 4) provide resources for the action plan task completion; 5) complete the template by listing the measurable, prioritized interventions with timelines and assigned personnel; and 6) track and monitor action plan progress on an ongoing basis.

9. What does an evaluation plan include for the data-driven action plan? (Step 6 of the PFOC)

    Answer: An evaluation plan includes the purpose of the evaluation, methods to measure progress, teams responsible for monitoring progress, how the evaluation results will be used to improve processes and decision-making, and how results will be shared.

Rationale for Implementation

After reading the chapter, ask the learners to test their understanding of the concepts with short answers.

1. Why is it important to create a comprehensive and compelling vision statement?

    Answer: A comprehensive and compelling vision statement helps to clarify direction, improve the ability to make informed decisions, and eliminate projects that are unnecessary and/or misaligned with the organization's mission and vision.

2. Why is it important to co-create and maintain team norms and a Civility Charter?

    Answer: The creation of team norms and a Civility Charter reinforces a commitment to communicate and interact with professionalism and respect. When disagreements arise, differences can be restricted to the issue itself, while continuing to respect the person with whom we disagree.

3. Why is accountability important to upholding team norms?

   Answer: Upholding team norms through accountability is vital to building a healthy work environment and fostering organizational civility. The absence of accountability is a strong predictor of failure in any shared decision-making model.

Application of the Concepts

Working in small groups, instruct learners to complete the following exercises.

1. Group Activity: Creating a Civility Vision Statement

At least a week prior to attending class, ask learners to find and bring a copy of their organization's mission, vision, and value statements to use during this activity. Encourage learners to consider their organization's mission, vision, and values statements and determine whether their organization has a corresponding healthy work environment and/or civility initiative in place. If one is in place, ask learners to bring the plan to class along with the other foundational statements. If their organization does not have a healthy work environment and/or civility initiative in place, encourage learners to consider how one might be implemented and how it can be aligned with the organizational vision, mission, and goals.

In small groups of four to five members, have each member briefly summarize their organizational statements. After all members have had an opportunity to describe their organizational statements, the group will select an organization among learners to use for creating a Civility Vision Statement. Review the selected organization's mission, vision, and values, and take 20 minutes to brainstorm about crafting a vision statement using the following formula:

Vision Statement Formula

The vision (purpose) of the civility and healthy workplace initiative is to _____ for (target population) _____ to fulfill the purpose of _____.

Upon completion of this statement, ask learners to identify specific strategies to share the civility vision with other members of the organization, and share the statement and communication strategies with the larger group. Learners should include at least one key takeaway point from this exercise that could help future efforts to create a Civility Vision Statement.

2. Group Activity: Co-Creating Team Norms

Using the same information from Activity 1, ask small groups of learners to co-create team norms relevant to the organization the group identified. Refer learners to pages 182 to 183 in the text for an example of team norms that could be included in a Civility Charter.

In small groups of four to five members, have learners co-create a list of team norms that are relevant to the organization's vision, mission, values, and commitment to its members. A spokesperson from each small group will share their answers to the following questions with the larger group of learners.

1. Share team norms created with the larger group.

2. Discuss why the team norms created are important for the organization.

3. Describe strategies for how members of the organization could be held accountable to upholding these team norms.

Reflection

Based on the experiences from the prior activities, have learners reflect on the process of creating team norms for an organization in small groups. Then have them answer the following questions:

1. Was the experience of creating norms as you expected? Why or why not?

2. Is there anything different you would do in the future when creating team norms? Describe what these actions would be if so.

Facilitator tip: Once learners have reflected on co-creating norms, have them share their insights with their work team and/or supervisor to glean additional perspectives and support.

References

Boswell, C., Opton, L., & Owen, D. C. (2017). Exploring shared governance for an academic nursing setting. *Journal of Nursing Education, 56*(4), 197–203. http://dx.doi.org.libproxy.boisestate.edu/10.3928/01484834-20170323-02

Bregman, P. (2016, January 11). The right way to hold people accountable. *Harvard Business Review*. https://hbr.org/2016/01/the-right-way-to-hold-people-accountable

Hess, R. G., Weaver, S. H., & Speroni, K. G. (2020). Shared governance during a pandemic. *Nurse Leader, 18*(5), 497–499. https://doi.org/10.1016/j.mnl.2020.05.008

Kotter, J. P. (1996). *Leading change.* Harvard Business Review Press.

Latham, J. R. (1995, April). Visioning: The concept, trilogy, and process. *Quality Progress, 28*(4), 65–68.

National Academies of Sciences, Engineering, and Medicine. (2019). *Taking action against clinician burnout: A systems approach to professional well-being.* https://doi.org/10.17226/25521

National Academy of Medicine (2022). *National plan for health workforce well-being and resilience.* https://nam.edu/initiatives/clinician-resilience-and-well-being/national-plan-for-health-workforce-well-being/

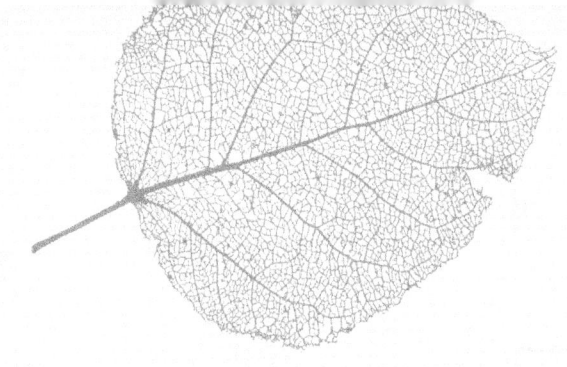

11

Securing Civility Into the Organizational Culture Through Policy Development

LEARNING OUTCOMES

- Explain the overall goal of a healthy work environment policy as a fundamental feature to shape and maintain a civil organizational culture.

- Discuss key factors to develop an effective policy to embed civility and healthy work environments into the organizational culture (Step 7 of the PFOC).

- Define and discuss the SMART policy to address and report incivility and to reward civility.

- Identify and discuss steps in the decision-making model for managing issues related to incivility.

- Describe the importance of using civility metrics to gauge employee performance and to use for hiring decisions.

Before You Begin

Chapter 11 highlights the importance of embedding civility into the organizational culture, policy development for fostering civility and healthy work environments (Step 7 of the Pathway for Fostering Organizational Civility [PFOC]), and a decision-making model for managing issues related to incivility in the work environment.

Everyone deserves, and likely desires, to work in a civil, healthy work environment where each person feels valued, respected, and appreciated. Employees at all levels of the organization have common social needs that need to be met for individuals and teams to thrive. These needs include feeling a sense of belonging, being respected and valued for their efforts and contributions, being aligned and committed to a shared vison and purpose, and participating in meaningful work. Creating a healthy work environment policy specifically addresses these important needs. In a recent McKinsey & Company report (Berlin et al., May 2022), nurses around the world said the most important factors keeping them in direct care roles included doing meaningful work, having a positive and engaging work environment, and feeling healthy and safe. Efforts to create a healthy work environment and feeling valued by a manager were ranked with high importance.

A well-constructed, confidential policy and procedure must be developed, implemented, and widely disseminated to foster a healthy work environment and embed positive changes into the organizational culture. Before facilitating learning activities associated with Chapter 11 content, it is helpful for facilitators to examine whether healthy work environment policies, procedures, or guidelines exist within their own organizations and, if so, when they were last reviewed and revised. Do they include specific step-by-step procedures to serve as a road map for reporting both acts of civility and incivility? How are acts of civility and other desired behaviors rewarded and celebrated? How are acts of incivility and other workplace aggressions managed? Is there a policy and/or decision-making process in place (e.g., SMART policy suggested by the author) to address complaints and reward desirable behaviors? If policies exist, do they reflect a commitment to diversity, equity, and inclusion? Are they easily accessible and widely disseminated? These are important aspects to consider prior to conducting class.

Next, think about your own experiences with incivility in the workplace. Have you or members of your team ever been accused of workplace bullying or other acts of workplace aggression? If so, what were the circumstances surrounding the accusations? How was the situation managed? Do you feel the situation was addressed in a fair and confidential manner? If you or a teammate have not been accused of workplace incivility or bullying, what measures have you taken to avoid accusations from occurring? What steps have you taken to ensure a healthy work environment?

Lastly, consider the hiring practices utilized within your department or organization. Does your team conduct structured group interviewing practices? What key questions are asked of interviewees during the interview process to vet for civility, character, teamwork, and collaboration? How are reference checks conducted, recorded, and acted upon? Do your interview practices include checking online profiles and social media posts? Does the interview team include questions about diversity, equity, and inclusion? How important are these characteristics to your team and organization?

In 2018, Wei et al, conducted a systematic review to describe the state of the science of nurse work environments in the United States. Because this review was conducted before the onset of the COVID-19 pandemic, facilitating class discussion on how the pandemic and its manifestations have influenced views on what constitutes a healthy nurse work environment has merit.

Facilitating learning activities on policy development and implementation can be challenging, especially when discussing sensitive topics such as addressing workplace incivility and other forms of aggression. However, the subject of policymaking bears deep discussion since it has the power to affect the systemic and long-term health of an organization. Discussion on policymaking enables learners to be thoughtfully engaged in ways to have a positive impact on workplace health. Understanding the rigors of policy development, implementation, and dissemination is an important skill set for all nurses and healthcare professionals.

Key Concepts

After reading the chapter, ask the learners to test their understanding of the concepts with short answers.

1. Describe the overall goal of a healthy work environment policy.

    Answer: The overall goal of a healthy work environment policy is to create a safe, collaborative work setting where all can thrive. A healthy work environment is a secure place where each individual feels supported and comfortable expressing diverse points of view, opinions, and beliefs.

2. Describe the key factors for effective policy development.

    Answer: There are several key factors to consider for effective policy development, including:

    - Ensuring strict confidentiality in the process for reporting uncivil behavior
    - Being specific about defining uncivil behavior and including a clear plan for addressing it
    - Ensuring fairness, consistency, and confidentiality, and including an incremental disciplinary approach when applicable, except in cases of egregious misconduct
    - Being comprehensive, easily accessible, and including specific step-by-step procedures
    - Containing several essential features, including: 1) a formal process for fostering a healthy work environment; 2) a fair, consistent, confidential procedure for defining and addressing workplace incivility; 3) a mechanism for reporting uncivil behavior and subsequent investigation of it; and 4) rewards for civil behavior and policy fulfillment

3. Identify and describe the five elements of the SMART policy.

   Answer: The five elements of the SMART policy are as follows:

   1. **S**ystem for confidential reporting: Reports about uncivil behavior are to be filed using a confidential, web-based reporting system. These reports include the following: 1) the reporter's contact information for follow-up purposes only; 2) information about the uncivil incident, such as its time, date, and location; 3) the impact of the uncivil incident; 4) the reporter's perception of and response to the uncivil incident; and 5) suggestions for following up about the uncivil incident.

   2. **M**anaging report information: Reports concerning uncivil behavior will be kept confidential and with need-to-know disclosure only to conduct a thorough investigation regarding the incident. The individual named in the report will be notified and provided an opportunity to meet with the individual filing the report and others designated to address and resolve the occurrence identified in the report.

   3. **A**ddressing incivility: If the report is validated, then a verbal warning will be provided to the person responsible for the uncivil behavior. Subsequent uncivil occurrences from the individual would result in a written Performance Improvement Plan (PIP), with behavioral requirements on a specified timeline. If no improvement in behavior occurs, then disciplinary action can be taken, such as suspension, temporary leave without pay, or termination.

   4. **R**ewarding civility: To reward civility, it would be helpful to include a similar confidential reporting system to document acts of civility and provide incentives, compensations, and/or rewards that the recipient desires. These data are also valuable to determine the success of the healthy work environment policy. Some low-cost, high-impact examples of rewarding civility include free lunch or dinner vouchers, movie tickets, gift cards, or a framed certificate.

   5. **T**racking and evaluating progress: The person designated for tracking effectiveness of the SMART policy will keep a record of each case and its outcome to generate a formal progress report. This report can be disseminated in aggregate to key members throughout the institution.

4. Describe steps one could take to address and manage a report of uncivil behavior in the workplace.

   Answer: To prepare for a meeting addressing a report of uncivil behavior from an individual, a supervisor could first schedule a meeting on a mutually agreed upon date, time, and location that is free from interruptions and distractions. Then, the supervisor responsible for facilitating the meeting should consider all perspectives about the incident before the meeting begins. During the meeting, the supervisor should maintain a neutral mindset while using active listening to attend to different perspectives of the incident. The supervisor is also encouraged to take notes and follow up with all parties regarding agreed upon solutions. If not resolved locally, the incident may need to be formally reported using the steps outlined in the healthy work environment policy.

5. Identify and describe the steps of the decision-making model for managing issues related to incivility.

    Answer: The steps of the decision-making model for managing issues related to incivility are as follows:

    1. Issue/concern: Civility Team receives written statement with detailed observations from person making the report.

    2. Discussion and review: Civility Team reviews written statement and evaluates the merit and impact of the issue/concern.

    3. Determine need for more information: Civility Team determines if additional information is needed, from whom, and within what time frame.

    4. Triage the issue/problem: If indicated, Civility Team refers issues/problems to most appropriate individual/team for resolution based on best practices, policy, and empirical evidence.

6. List some questions interviewees could ask job applicants about issues of diversity, equity, and inclusion as related to civility.

    Answer: The following five questions about diversity, equity, and inclusion related to civility could be asked of interviewees:

    1. Describe a situation where you created an inclusive environment for all members of your (team, unit, class, organization). Describe the situation, the actions you took, and the outcome. What lessons did you learn from the experience?

    2. What diversity, equity, and inclusion courses have you completed? How have you applied what you learned in the workplace? Give specific examples.

    3. Give two or three examples of how your work life has been enhanced by exposure to diverse people, places, or experiences.

    4. How have the perspectives of underrepresented groups impacted your professional career? Provide one or two examples.

    5. What specific actions have you taken to create civility and an inclusive work environment?

Rationale for Implementation

After reading the chapter, ask the learners to test their understanding of the concepts with short answers.

1. Why is it important to create a healthy work environment policy?

    Answer: The overall goal of a healthy work environment policy is to create a safe, collaborative work setting where all can thrive—a secure place where each individual feels supported and comfortable expressing diverse and differing points of view, opinions, and beliefs.

2. Why is it important to hire for civility and link civility to performance metrics?

    Answer: Taking a proactive approach to hire for civility helps avoid bringing incivility and other toxic behaviors into the workplace. Group interviewing can be helpful in screening candidates because group interviewing engages multiple perspectives when considering potential candidates.

Application of the Concepts

Working in small groups, instruct learners to complete the following exercises.

1. Group Activity: Healthy Work Environment Policy Critique

Ask learners to reread the healthy work environment policy exemplar on pages 195 to 199. Then, have learners gather into small groups to critique the policy using the questions listed below. Next, ask learners to identify items or content they might add, delete, or modify when considering a healthy work environment policy for their specific organization. After answering questions and identifying any additions, deletions, or modifications, have learners re-convene as a larger group and share at least three key takeaways from their small group discussion.

Policy critique: Using a scale from 1 to 4 (1 = strongly disagree, 2 = disagree, 3 = agree, 4 = strongly agree), rate the level of agreement for the following questions. Then discuss your ratings and rationale within your small group.

1. To what extent does the policy meet the overall objective of creating and sustaining a healthy work environment to transform the organizational culture?

2. To what extent are the policy purpose, policy statement, and commitment to civility well defined and clearly stated for all members of the organization?

3. To what extent are the list of shared values and statement on incivility and other workplace aggressions relevant to fostering a healthy work environment?

4. To what extent are the examples of incivility and other workplace aggressions and the examples of desired behaviors relevant to fostering a healthy work environment?

5. To what extent are the procedure and reporting statements clearly stated for all members of the organization?

6. To what extent does the policy promote systemic change and long-term sustainability?

2. Group Activity: Civility Conversation Role-Play Between Manager and Reported Employee

Ask learners to assemble into small groups and identify a real or potential uncivil scenario that could occur in their workplace. Then, using the information contained on pages 202 to 203 ("Civility Conversations for Managers and Supervisors"), ask learners to write a script based on the scenario. The script includes the role of a "manager" and the role of an "employee" who will be meeting to discuss a complaint that has been filed against the employee accusing them of a serious act of workplace aggression. While still in their small groups, learners will identify group members to play the roles of "manager" and "employee." Suggest to learners that the PAAIL method (first introduced in Chapter 5 and revisited on page 204) and/or other evidence-based frameworks contained in Chapter 5 provide approaches to leading a civility conversation. After completing the script of the uncivil encounter, learners will role-play the scenario for the larger group. Facilitators will lead a debriefing session after the role-play to identify what went well and what could be improved.

Facilitator-led debriefing questions:

1. **For actors:** What was it like to be part of this experience? What thoughts and/or feelings were evoked?

2. **For observers:** What was it like to observe the experience? What did you see? What did you hear?

3. **For all** participants and observers:
    a. How would you describe the conversation?
    b. What went well, and what would you do again?
    c. What was most effective about the conversation?
    d. What might be done differently next time?
    e. How might you apply what you have learned in your clinical practice?

Reflection

Ask learners to reflect on whether their specific organization has implemented a policy to foster civility and a healthy work environment. Then have them answer the following questions:

1. Does a healthy work environment policy exist?
2. If so, does it include a confidential, step-by-step procedure to serve as a road map for reporting both acts of civility and incivility?
3. Does the policy reflect a commitment to diversity, equity, and inclusion?
4. Is the policy easily accessible and widely disseminated?
5. If a healthy work environment policy does not exist in your organization, what steps might you take to assemble and lead a team to develop and implement a healthy work environment policy?

Facilitator tip: Once learners have reflected on policy development for creating and sustaining healthy work environments, have them share their insights with their work team and/or supervisor to glean additional perspectives and support.

References

Berlin, G., Essick, C., LaPointe, M., & Lyons, F. (May 2022). *Around the world, nurses say meaningful work keeps them going.* McKinsey & Company report. https://www.mckinsey.com/industries/healthcare-systems-and-services/our-insights/around-the-world-nurses-say-meaningful-work-keeps-them-going

Wei, H., Sewell, K. A., Woody, G., & Rose, M. A. (2018). The state of the science of nurse work environments in the United States: A systematic review. *International Journal of Nursing Sciences, 5*(3), 287–300. https://doi.org/10.1016/j.ijnss.2018.04.010

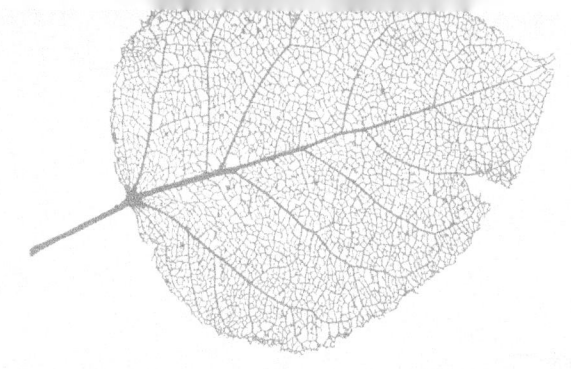

12

Celebrating Civility: A Powerful Engine to Uplift and Transform the Profession

LEARNING OUTCOMES

- Identify methods to consolidate gains and build momentum as part of Step 8 of the PFOC.
- Describe methods to expand the civility initiative and sustain organizational transformation as part of Step 8 of the PFOC.
- Discuss the importance of celebrating civility in an organization of nursing and healthcare professionals.
- Explain the importance of hope and optimism to transform nursing and healthcare professions.

Before You Begin

Chapter 12 highlights ways to consolidate gains, celebrate civility, expand the Healthy Work Environment (HWE) initiative (Step 8 of the Pathway for Fostering Organizational Civility [PFOC]), and reap hope and optimism to transform the healthcare professions. When preparing to facilitate learning experiences on these important topics, consider ways that your department or organization celebrates short- and long-term wins and meaningfully recognizes employees and/or learners. Meaningful recognition is one of the American Association of Critical-Care Nurses (AACN, 2016) standards for achieving a healthy work environment—this means acknowledging individual and collective contributions throughout the organization in significant ways. Think about ways that meaningful recognition is expressed in your workplace. Have there been times when you or a colleague or classmate received meaningful recognition? If so, how were you or your colleague or classmate recognized? What feelings and thoughts were evoked when you were meaningfully recognized? How did meaningful recognition affect others and contribute to a healthy work or learning environment?

In a similar vein, the author makes a case for rewarding civility and other desired behaviors to consolidate gains and fuel momentum for ongoing organizational transformation. The author further asserts that rewarding civility contributes to increased morale, job satisfaction, and collegiality; positive recruitment and retention of employees; increased job satisfaction; and continued momentum toward the change effort. With these statements in mind, consider whether civility and collegiality are rewarded on a daily and ongoing basis in your workplace. If so, what impact have these rewards had on fostering and sustaining a healthy work and/or learning environment? Think about ways that you have recognized and rewarded others for their achievements, contributions, and acts of civility. What was the impact of your recognition of others?

Chapter 12 also details Step 8 of the PFOC, which includes expanding and building momentum for the civility initiative. This expansion includes rotation and replacement of Civility Team members; identifying individual, team, and organizational accomplishments; reviewing progression and assessment of the data-driven action plan; and sharing lessons learned. These efforts are done to determine the effectiveness of the civility initiative and to embed changes into the organizational culture. Facilitators are urged to familiarize themselves with strategies to evaluate action plans and ways to ensure sustainability.

AACN's (2016) six essential standards provide evidence-based guidelines to build and sustain healthy work environments. AACN contends that the healthiest work environments integrate all six standards. Harmon et al. (2018) recommended that schools of nursing adopt the six AACN standards as well as incorporating a seventh standard of self-care since stress can impede an individual's ability to function well. In addition to meaningful recognition (noted earlier in this section), facilitators should familiarize themselves with all six AACN standards and include self-care as a seventh standard when discussing standards for creating and sustaining healthy work and learning environments with learners. The seven standards include:

- Skilled communication
- True collaboration
- Effective decision-making
- Appropriate staffing
- Meaningful recognition
- Authentic leadership
- Self-care

Chapter 12 also focuses on achieving a view of the future balanced with optimism and realism. As a facilitator, consider your view of the future. Has your level of optimism declined or expanded in the aftermath of the COVID pandemic? Do you believe there are benefits to being optimistic? How can we balance optimism with the undeniable realities of heightened levels of stress, anxiety, moral distress, and burnout that healthcare professionals are facing? How does one stay optimistic when confronted with these and other challenges? How can we achieve tragic optimism and find meaning and purpose amid these very real challenges and setbacks?

Key Concepts

After reading the chapter, ask the learners to test their understanding of the concepts with short answers.

1. Identify methods to consolidate gains and build momentum as part of Step 8 of the PFOC.

   Answer: Consolidating gains and building momentum can be achieved through celebrating civility throughout an organization. Methods to celebrate civility include: 1) acknowledging the efforts of employees to foster civility throughout the workday; 2) writing a personal note of thanks to a deserving person, their manager, or their family member; 3) monthly birthday parties to acknowledge every employee whose birthday occurs that month; 4) distributing small tokens of appreciation (i.e., coffee/tea mugs and T-shirts); 5) smiling and saying "thank you"; 6) including a note of recognition in a departmental email; 7) providing a signed certificate of appreciation; 8) creating a formal program in the organization to reward civility; and 9) hosting a civility summit in the organization to showcase individual and collective acts of civility.

2. Discuss processes to expand the civility initiative as a part of sustaining organizational transformation for a healthier, more civil work environment.

   Answer: The process of expanding the civility initiative includes maintaining and building sustained interest in the effort while also inviting new members to join efforts to create and sustain a healthier work environment. While some members of the Civility Team may remain on the team, others may rotate onto the team to continue facilitating the change process to implement the healthy work environment initiative. As part of the process to bring new members onto the Civility Team, it is important to discuss individual, team, and organizational accomplishments; review progression and assessment of the data-driven action plan; and share lessons learned. Newly onboarded members of the Civility Team could also benefit from a workshop or off-campus retreat to provide new members with an expanded view of the healthy work environment initiative and how it can be improved and evaluated in the future.

3. What is *tragic optimism*, and why is it important to informing hope and optimism to transform health professions?

    Answer: Tragic optimism can be described as optimism in the face of tragedy (Mead et al., 2021) and places an emphasis on achieving a hopeful outlook despite distress and suffering. According to Frankl, "Tragic optimism means that one is, and remains, optimistic in spite of the tragic triad, which consists of those aspects of human existence which may be circumscribed by: 1) pain; 2) guilt; and 3) death" (Frankl, 1984, p. 139). Looking at situations through the lens of tragic optimism acknowledges the distressing realities of life while also acknowledging life's importance and meaning under all conditions, therefore informing and building purpose and hope in health professions.

4. What is *toxic positivity*, and why is it important to avoid during efforts to foster hope and optimism to transform health professions?

    Answer: Toxic positivity can be described as unrelenting optimism that fails to acknowledge hardships or recognize the true, sometimes distressing nature of a situation. Avoiding the unpleasant realties of a situation can prevent growth from both the good and detrimental aspects of a circumstance. Therefore, it is important to acknowledge the good and unpleasant aspects of a circumstance to foster positive developments in health professions.

Rationale for Implementation

After reading the chapter, ask the learners to test their understanding of the concepts with short answers.

1. Why is it important to celebrate civility in an organization?

    Answer: Rewarding civil acts fuels momentum for ongoing organizational transformation and contributes to heightened levels of morale, job satisfaction, and collegiality. Celebrating civility is critically important because doing so can motivate employees at all levels of the organization to continue contributing to a culture of civility.

2. Why is it important to expand the civility initiative?

   Answer: Expanding the civility initiative to include other members of the organization to participate on the Civility Team can help build momentum to continue and advance the civility initiative throughout the organization.

Application of the Concepts

Working in small groups, instruct learners to complete the following exercises.

1. Research & Group Activity: Celebrating Civility: A Tiered Approach

Have learners bring their laptop, tablet, or smartphone to class. This learning exercise combines an internet search with a small group activity. Ask learners to conduct an internet search of ways to celebrate or reward civility and other desired workplace behaviors. The search includes celebrations or rewards that are no cost, low cost, and higher cost. Have learners take notes on the results of their search and identify at least one civility celebration or reward for each level (no cost, low cost, higher cost). Once the search is completed and notes have been taken, have learners assemble into small groups and ask them to share their findings with group members. Ask each small group to select one celebration or reward for each cost level and describe how they would integrate the celebration or reward into the work or learning environment. If time permits, have learners share their findings with the larger group.

1. For each cost tier (no cost, low cost, and higher cost), evaluate the pros and cons for designing and implementing the civility celebration ideas found through an internet search.
2. Select the top idea for each cost tier to share with a larger group of learners.
3. Describe the rationale for selecting each idea considering the cost tier and the main motivation for these selections.
4. Discuss the most appealing aspects about celebration ideas found at the three cost levels.
5. Discuss how you would advocate for enacting these ideas in your workplace.

2. Case Study Group Activity: Navigating and Sustaining Interest in the Civility Initiative

Have learners gather in groups of four to five or fewer depending on the group's size. In a 30-minute time frame, encourage learners to discuss the following scenario from multiple perspectives, including the individual, workgroup, and larger organizational perspective. For example, the individual perspective could be from Professor Gomez's point of view, as well as other members of the Civility Team and organizational leaders. Encourage learners to form their response to the first question posed from Professor Gomez's perspective and then to shift their focus to thinking about navigating changes in the Civility Team from a larger, organizational perspective. Once learners have finished their discussions in their small groups, ask them to re-convene and share their most salient points of discussion with the large group.

Scenario

For the past year, Professor Gomez has been a major contributor for the School of Nursing's Civility Team. As a founding member of the Civility Team, Professor Gomez has invested significant time and effort to ensure its success. The Civility Team's progress has been substantial, with several notable accomplishments, including completing a baseline comprehensive assessment and plan for creating and sustaining a civil work environment, the development and implementation of an organizational civility policy to address uncivil behavior, and the development and implementation of a web-based confidential reporting system for tracking and addressing uncivil incidents. Professor Gomez implemented a pre-post survey to measure and document the effect of the Civility Team's interventions and found that, overall, faculty and staff morale about promoting a civil environment has improved as correlated to the Civility Team's efforts. Although Professor Gomez has been a strong contributing member of the Civility Team, she is concerned that her recently funded research project will require her to devote more time and effort to research and less time to Civility Team responsibilities. Professor Gomez has a strong desire for the Civility Team to succeed and for their efforts to remain a priority in the School of Nursing. When Professor Gomez communicates her need to redirect her focus to research, she discovers that another Civility Team member has similar competing demands. As the team problem-solves the situation, they realize that a process is needed to expand the civility initiative and bring new members onto the Civility Team in an ongoing manner.

Considering this case, think about and answer the following prompts:

1. How could Professor Gomez best communicate her needs to the Civility Team in a manner that is respectful to the team and to herself?
2. What processes could be put in place to monitor and reward time spent on the Civility Team as part of the organization's vision to create and sustain a healthy work environment?
3. In addition to time, what other resources may be needed to expand the civility initiative?
4. How might the organizational bylaws assist in bringing new members onto the Civility Team?

Reflection

Stories engage and activate emotion and connect us to one another. Telling a simple, powerful, relevant story breathes life and relevance into everyday life. When we share stories, we make meaning of and provide context for understanding our own and others' lived experiences. For this reflection exercise, have learners begin by rereading the quote on page 223 of the text: "We are writing history right now, and we hold the pen. We are and can be the heroes in this story!" Have learners take 10 to 15 minutes to compose a story from their life or work experience that sheds a positive light on how navigating and overcoming challenges can lead to a positive and productive future.

Facilitator tip: Once learners have written their stories, have them share their stories with a friend, family member, neighbor, coworker, classmate, or other person of choice.

References

American Association of Critical-Care Nurses. (2016). *AACN standards for establishing and sustaining healthy work environments: A journey to excellence* (2nd ed.). http://www.aacn.org/WD/HWE/Docs/HWEStandards.pdf

Frankl, V. (1984). *Man's search for meaning*. Simon & Schuster.

Harmon, R. B., DeGennaro, G., Norling, M., Kennedy, C., & Fontaine, D. (2018). Implementing healthy work environment standards in an academic workplace: An update. *Journal of Professional Nursing, 34*(1), 20–24.

Mead, J. P., Fisher, Z., Tree, J. J., Wong, P., & Kemp, A. H. (2021). Protectors of wellbeing during the COVID-19 pandemic: Key roles for gratitude and tragic optimism in a UK-based cohort. *Frontiers in Psychology, 12*, 647951. https://doi.org/10.3389/fpsyg.2021.647951

www.ingramcontent.com/pod-product-compliance
Lightning Source LLC
Chambersburg PA
CBHW060234240426
43671CB00016B/2935